Your Personal Fitness Trainer

David H. Bass

Ziff-Davis Press
Emeryville, California

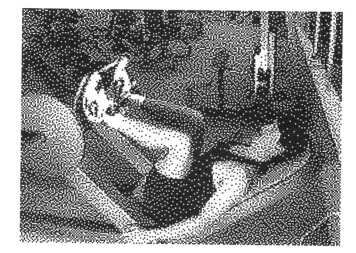

Editors	Deborah Craig and Cheryl Holzaepfel
Assistant Editor	Stephanie Raney
CD-ROM Reviewer	Tony Jonick
Project Coordinator	Barbara Dahl
Proofreader	Carol Burbo
Cover Design and Illustration	Regan Honda
Book Design	Laura Lamar/MAX, San Francisco
Technical Illustration	Dave Feasey and Sarah Ishida
Word Processing	Howard Blechman
Page Layout	Bruce Lundquist

Ziff-Davis Press books are produced on a Macintosh computer system with the following applications: FrameMaker®, Microsoft® Word, QuarkXPress®, Adobe Illustrator®, Adobe Photoshop®, Adobe Streamline™, MacLink®*Plus*, Aldus® FreeHand™, Collage Plus™.

If you have comments or questions or would like to receive a free catalog, call or write:
Ziff-Davis Press
5903 Christie Avenue
Emeryville, CA 94608
1-800-688-0448

ISBN 1-56276-312-1

Manufactured in the United States of America
10 9 8 7 6 5 4 3 2 1

TABLE OF CONTENTS

ACKNOWLEDGMENTS

I would like to thank Sean Morgan, Sam Miller, Neil Pasaro, Markus Lobl, Guy Loundagin, James Campodonico, my family and friends, and most of all my wife, Susan Woolley, for all their help and inspiration during the creation of this book and CD-ROM. Without all of them, this dream would never have become a reality.

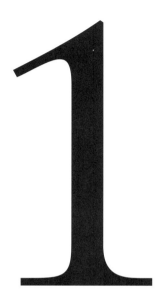

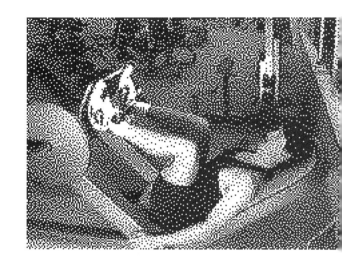

Getting Off on the Right Foot

Why a Fitness Program?

What Are Your Health and Fitness Goals?

Sticking with Your Fitness Program

THIS CHAPTER WILL GET YOU OFF ON THE RIGHT FOOT BY EXPLAINING JUST what a fitness program is and how you can benefit from one. Once you understand what you stand to gain, and see how potentially easy a basic fitness program can be, you'll probably feel less intimidated by the prospect (if you're on the out-of-shape side) or even positively enthusiastic about the whole idea (if you're in better shape). The chapter will also give you some sense of how to assess your health and fitness goals so you can decide not only where you are but where you want to go in fitness terms. Finally, you'll learn some strategies for sticking with your program. These techniques will help you make fitness a regular, and even enjoyable, part of your life, instead of an unpleasant chore or something that you force yourself to do for a week or two as a result of yet another new year's resolution.

Why a Fitness Program?

Fitness can mean different things to different people. One dictionary describes "fitness" as being physically and mentally sound. You can think of fitness as maintaining and improving the quality of your physical and mental health.

One of the best ways to improve your health is to begin a physical fitness program. A good program should include strength training with weights, cardiovascular exercise, stretching, and a proper diet. Carrying out a fitness program that includes these four components will help to increase your muscular strength and endurance, your flexibility, and your cardiovascular capacity, and improve your nutrition. Performing these forms of exercise regularly is the most efficient way to maintain and improve your fitness level.

Quality of Life

Improving your physical fitness levels will also improve your quality of life. Embarking on a fitness program can be a major change in lifestyle. Although you shouldn't make fitness an obsession, you should incorporate exercise into your schedule at least three times per week for 20 to 60 minutes per exercise session.

This amount of exercise may seem like too much of a commitment for certain dedicated couch potatoes. If you fall into this category, it may help to think small at the beginning. Try to keep in mind that you can improve your health greatly by exercising just a small amount, as long as you do so regularly. In fact, it's much better to exercise in small doses, but consistently, than it is to exercise in long but infrequent sessions. For example, it's better to walk for 15 to 20 minutes every two or three days than to run 5 miles once a month.

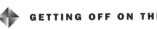

As mentioned, once you begin exercising you'll discover that it improves your quality of life. Obviously, quality of life can have different meanings for different people. Among other things, it can mean the following:

Having More Energy   A fitness program enhances your level of energy because exercise increases your basal metabolic rate over time. Your *basal metabolic rate* is the natural amount of calories you burn at rest throughout the day. As you improve your fitness level, your body will become more efficient, and you will have more energy throughout the day. Although it may seem paradoxical, rather than making you tired, exercise will actually provide you with extra energy in the long run.

Getting Stronger   A fitness program enhances your muscle strength and endurance because strength training increases your muscle mass and skeletal density. As you improve your fitness level, your body will become stronger, with benefits that will last the rest of your life. Increased muscle mass and skeletal density not only facilitate certain tasks—such as lifting groceries or carrying a suitcase—but may also help prevent injuries.

Losing Pounds of Body Fat   A fitness program enhances your body's ability to burn fat and calories. In addition, cardiovascular exercise increases your expenditure of calories. Expending calories while you're exercising will help remove inches from your body and eventually help you lose overall pounds of fat.

Breathing More Easily   A fitness program can make you breathe more easily. Cardiovascular exercise increases your lungs' capacity for oxygen, improving your entire respiratory system in the process.

Improving Your Motor Skills   A fitness program increases your muscular strength, cardiovascular endurance, and flexibility. These qualities help improve the motor skills you need to excel in an activity or sport.

Decreasing Your Risk of Disease and Infection   A fitness program heightens your body's ability to fight disease and infection. For example, cardiovascular exercise helps decrease your resting blood pressure level, which in turn decreases your risk of heart attack.

Decreasing Your Risk of Injury   A fitness program enhances your body's muscular strength, cardiovascular endurance, and flexibility. These qualities, in turn, make it less likely that you'll injure yourself while participating in a sport, carrying out fitness exercises, or performing daily activities such as lifting objects, walking, running to catch a bus, and the like.

Decreasing Your Daily Stress Levels   A fitness program increases your body's level of eustress, or positive stress, and decreases your body's level of distress, or negative stress. Positive stress can lead to physical and mental excitement, delight, and creativity. Negative stress usually triggers feelings such as fear, pressure, worry, or disappointment. Managing stress is the key to overcoming and learning from both the positive and negative situations in our daily lives.

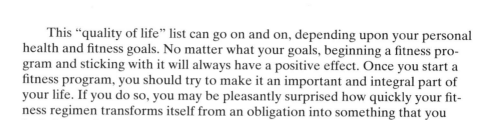

This "quality of life" list can go on and on, depending upon your personal health and fitness goals. No matter what your goals, beginning a fitness program and sticking with it will always have a positive effect. Once you start a fitness program, you should try to make it an important and integral part of your life. If you do so, you may be pleasantly surprised how quickly your fitness regimen transforms itself from an obligation into something that you look forward to because it helps you work out the kinks and tensions that you accumulate from day to day.

What Are Your Health and Fitness Goals?

Before you leap headlong into a fitness program, it's a good idea to take stock of your goals. What exactly do you want to get out of your fitness program? What's the best way to achieve your health and fitness aims? This section encourages you to ask yourself some of these questions, and helps you determine where you can find some answers.

Muscular Strength

One reason to start a fitness program is to increase your muscular strength, or to improve your muscles' overall strength and speed during an exercise or activity. To build up your muscular strength, you need to lift increasingly heavy volumes of weight with minimal repetitions during a specific exercise. For example, if you're performing a bench press, you might increase the resistance (weight volume) from 120 pounds for 10 repetitions during the first set to 150 pounds for 7 repetitions during the second set.

 If you want to improve your muscular strength level, the American College of Sports Medicine recommends that you perform strength training exercises three days per week for a minimum of 20 minutes. For further details on improving your muscular strength, click on the Personal Fitness Training Program icon in the CD-ROM's icon menu, then select Strength Training.

Muscular Endurance

Another reason to start a fitness program is to build up your muscular endurance, or your muscles' ability to withstand fatigue during exercise or other activities. To increase your muscular endurance, you need to lift light to moderate volumes of weight with maximal repetitions during a specific exercise. For example, if you're performing a bench press, you might increase the number of repetitions per set while lifting a consistent weight of 120 pounds. (In other words, you're increasing the repetitions without increasing the weight, while in muscular strength tests you're increasing the weight without increasing the repetitions.)

If you want to improve your muscular endurance level, the American College of Sports Medicine recommends that you perform strength training exercises three days per week for a minimum of 20 minutes. For further details on improving your muscular endurance, click on the Personal Fitness Training Program icon in the CD-ROM's icon menu, then select Strength Training.

Aerobic Improvement

You might also decide to start a fitness program to get into better aerobic shape. You can begin a cardiovascular training program to increase your level of maximal oxygen intake (aerobic or VO2 capacity). Aerobic exercise involves performing a low-to-moderate-intensity activity which supplies a sufficient level of energy and oxygen to the working muscles of the body for an extended period of time.

If you to want to improve your aerobic endurance level, the American College of Sports Medicine recommends that you perform a consistent regimen of cardiovascular exercise three days per week for a minimum of 20 minutes. For further details about improving your cardiorespiratory system, click on the Personal Fitness Training Program icon in the CD-ROM's icon menu, then select Cardiovascular Training.

Body Fat and Weight Loss

Many people embark on fitness programs to lose weight. The key to losing body fat and body weight is to understand that loss of body fat is more important than loss of overall body weight. If you lose body fat, you reduce your risk of coronary artery disease; losing overall body weight doesn't necessarily reduce your risk of coronary artery disease. If you diet without exercising, you may lose body weight without losing body fat. Conversely, if you exercise, you may lose body fat without losing body weight. In other words, you shouldn't be discouraged if regular exercise doesn't immediately begin decreasing your body weight. The exercise should be decreasing your body fat level, and improving your health in the process.

Before beginning any health and fitness program, you should understand that the amount of body fat and body weight that you lose depends in part on your body type. In addition, your daily dietary habits and your physical activity level affect your body fat and body weight levels. For further information on body fat level and weight loss, refer to Chapter 3, which explains how to obtain a body composition test and what the results mean. For further details on body fat and weight loss, click on the Nutrition and Personal Fitness Training Program icons in the CD-ROM's icon menu. You should also read through Chapter 6, which discusses nutrition.

Flexibility Enhancement

Stretching should be a part of any fitness program. Stretching increases the range of motion of both your muscles and joints. Increasing your flexibility in this way helps you avoid injury. It also elongates your muscle groups, and greater muscle length helps to produce greater muscle size and muscle strength. For this reason, you should incorporate stretching exercises into any strength training and any cardiovascular training program. For further details on improving your flexibility, click on the Personal Fitness Training Program icon in the CD-ROM's icon menu, then select Stretching and Flexibility.

Sticking with Your Fitness Program

You have already learned a bit about the mental and physical benefits of a fitness program. Despite these pluses, however, many people have trouble sticking with their program. It's common for people to begin an exercise program and quit within the first few weeks or months because they lack motivation. This section includes some suggestions that should help you stick with your fitness program. Although old habits of physical inactivity may die hard, putting out the effort to stay with your program is certainly worthwhile. As we've mentioned, once you get into the fitness habit, you may find yourself looking forward to your fitness program with pleasure rather than with dread.

The Buddy System

Using the "buddy system" simply means having a friend or relative participate in a fitness program with you. Having someone else to encourage and motivate you while you exercise will go a long way toward helping you stick with your fitness program longer. Working out with a buddy is also a good way of making strength, endurance, and cardiovascular exercises more safe.

A Personal Fitness Trainer

An advanced form of the buddy system is working with a personal fitness trainer. A personal fitness trainer can educate you, motivate you, and manage your fitness program. Look for a personal fitness trainer who has a degree in exercise science or physical education and who is certified through the American College of Sports Medicine, the National Sports Performance Association, or the National Strength and Conditioning Association. Such a trainer will be a qualified professional who can craft a fitness program that is tailored to meet your health and fitness needs.

Varying Your Workout

If you vary your workout, changing the sequence of your exercises, the number of sets you perform, the number of repetitions, and the weight that you use for each exercise, you stimulate your muscles in different ways. "Muscle stimulation" refers to an increase in the size, strength, and endurance of the muscle.

You can stimulate your muscles in any one of the following ways:

You can change the number of repetitions and the sets you perform for each muscle group. For example, you could perform three sets of 10 repetitions for four weeks with a moderate weight (60 to 80% of your one-repetition maximum), and then switch to three sets of eight repetitions for four weeks with a heavy level of weight volume (80 to 100% of your one-repetition maximum).

You can change the order in which you exercise the muscle groups that you are strength training. For instance, you could train your chest muscles before training your back muscles and then switch to training your back muscles before your chest muscles.

You can exercise with weights first and perform cardiovascular exercise afterwards. This may help to increase muscle stimulation because your body will have more caloric energy to expend during the weight training portion of your fitness program.

For more in-depth information about set selection, repetition selection, and weight volume, consult the personal fitness training section of the CD-ROM. For more information on improving your muscular strength and endurance, click on the Personal Fitness Training Program icon in the CD-ROM's icon menu, then select Strength Training.

Avoiding the "Overuse Syndrome"

The overuse syndrome occurs when your joints and muscles are consistently stressed with resistance or motion in the same sequence for an extended period of time. An example would be continuous humerus (upper arm bone) compression into the shoulder joint caused by performing the bench press exercise with a consistent weight volume and then performing the incline bench press exercise with a consistent weight volume.

If you constantly repeat this same chest exercise sequence—performing the same exercise, the same number of sets, and an identical number of repetitions with an unchanging weight volume—for an extended period of time, you increase your risk of injury and decrease your potential for strength improvement and muscle stimulation in your chest muscles. Instead, make sure to vary the weights that you use and the sequence in which you perform your exercises.

Fighting Boredom

It's not out of the question that you might eventually become bored with your fitness program. Exercising the exact same way for an extended period of time can certainly become monotonous. One of the best ways to keep from getting bored with your fitness program is to consistently change your exercises every three to four weeks. This is a great way keep your fitness program interesting and fun. It can also help to nip other problems—such as overuse syndrome—in the bud.

Reevaluating and Remotivating

It's important to measure your progress throughout your fitness program. If you evaluate your fitness levels every three to four months, you'll get a concrete picture of how your fitness program is working. Seeing the improvements in your fitness level can also motivate you to continue your fitness program. Please refer to Chapter 3 or to the "Getting Started" section in the CD-ROM for further information about measuring your fitness levels.

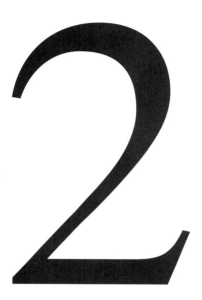

2

Equipment for Keeping Fit

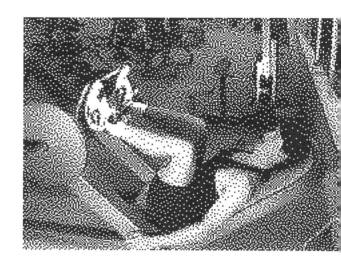

Selecting a Fitness Center

Designing a Home Gym

T'S IMPORTANT TO EXERCISE IN AN ENVIRONMENT THAT IS SAFE, PLEASANT, and properly equipped. When selecting a fitness center, first check it out carefully, making sure it meets your needs before you make a final decision to join. Among other things, you should look for sufficient equipment in good repair, a well-trained and courteous staff, and aerobic or other fitness classes that suit your ability level and your schedule. When setting up a home gym, you should make sure to select the equipment that is appropriate for you. This chapter teaches you a bit about both of these things. Throughout, keep in mind that you should exercise in the environment that you prefer. If you enjoy working out in a neighborhood fitness center, by all means do your workouts there. If you prefer to exercise at home, that's fine, too. Some people even like to divide their workout between home and a fitness center. It doesn't matter much where you exercise, but it's critical that you exercise regularly, and that you exercise safely.

Selecting a Fitness Center

When choosing a fitness center, you should try ahead of time to evaluate the fitness center facility, the staff, the equipment, and any available classes and programs to make sure the center will adequately meet your requirements.

The Fitness Center Facility

If possible, try to select a fitness center that is associated with the International Health, Racquet, and Sportsclub Association (IHRSA). This association is a leader in the fitness industry for recognizing quality fitness facilities. IHRSA offers membership to facilities throughout the world. All IHRSA membership clubs have reciprocity privileges, which means that if you belong to one such gym, you are free to work out at any other. This can be particularly handy if you travel a lot for business, or if you like to keep up with your workouts when you go on vacation.

The American College of Sports Medicine has developed guidelines for evaluating a safe and quality fitness center, and they have a handbook that spells out what a fitness center should have in terms of equipment, staffing, programming, and operations. When looking for the right fitness center facility, make sure that it meets the following criteria:

- It should have clean locker rooms and lavatories.

- The staff should be courteous and service oriented and should be certified (see below).

- The fitness equipment and aerobics class area should be well-maintained.

- The fitness center must be convenient to your home or work.

The Fitness Center Staff

If you select a member of the fitness staff to administer your personal fitness training program, he or she should possess

- A bachelors, masters, or doctoral degree in exercise science or physical education.

- A current continuing education certification credential from one or more of the following health and fitness professional organizations:

  - The American College of Sports Medicine (ACSM)

  - The National Sports Performance Association (NSPA)

  - The National Strength and Conditioning Association (NSCA)

  - The American Council on Exercise (ACE)

Fitness Center Equipment

You must have access to the proper equipment in order to begin your fitness program. Your fitness center should have the strength training and cardiovascular training equipment listed in the following tables. If you're not sure how to recognize the various pieces of equipment, ask a member of the fitness center for a guided tour, having him or her point out which machines the center has, what they're for, and how to use them. Note that some smaller gyms may not have all the equipment listed for exercising the same sets of muscle groups.

Lower-Body Strength Training Equipment	Focused Muscle Groups Used
Leg press sled	Entire lower body
45-degree seated leg press	Entire lower body
Squat rack/cage	Entire lower body
Smith press machine	Entire lower body
Multistation unit	Entire lower body
Multi-hip machine	Hips, adductors, abductors, gluteals
Hip adduction machine	Hips, adductors, abductors, gluteals

Hip abduction machine	Hips, adductors, abductors, gluteals
Cable column unit	Hips, adductors, abductors, gluteals
Leg extension machine	Quadriceps
Leg curl machine	Hamstrings
Seated calf raise machine	Calves
Standing calf raise machine	Calves

Upper-Body Strength Training Equipment	**Focused Muscle Groups Used**
Assisted dip and chin up machine	Entire upper body
Smith press machine	Entire upper body
Adjustable incline/flat bench	Entire upper body
Cable column unit	Entire upper body
Cable crossover machine	Entire upper body
Multistation unit	Entire upper body
Chest press machine	Chest, shoulders, triceps
Chest fly machine or peck deck	Chest, shoulders
Incline chest press machine	Chest, shoulders, triceps
Flat Olympic bench	Chest, shoulders, triceps
Incline Olympic bench	Chest, shoulders, triceps
Lat pull-down machine	Upper back, biceps, forearms
Seated row machine	Upper back, biceps, forearms
Cable row/low pull machine	Upper/lower back, biceps, forearms

Back extension machine	Lower back, hips
45-degree back extension	Lower back, hips
Shoulder press machine	Shoulders, triceps
Side lateral deltoid machine	Shoulders
Rear deltoid machine	Shoulders
Triceps extension machine	Triceps
Dip/triceps push-down machine	Triceps, chest
Biceps curl machine	Biceps
Preacher curl bench	Biceps
Abdominal crunch board	Abdominals, hips, lower back

Free-Weight Equipment for the Upper Body and Lower Body

Olympic bar

E-Z curl bar

Cable bar handles (straight and curved)

Single cable handle

Single cable ankle straps

Free-weight plates (2.5 lbs., 5 lbs., 10 lbs., 25 lbs., 35 lbs., 45 lbs.)

Dumbbells (1 lb., 2 lbs., 3 lbs., 5 lbs. 8 lbs., 10 lbs., 12 lbs., 15 lbs., 20 lbs.–100 lbs.)

Cardiovascular Training Equipment	Focused Muscle Groups Used
Stair-climbing machine	Entire lower body
Stationary cycle	Entire lower body
Recumbent cycle	Entire lower body
Computerized stair-climbing machine	Entire lower body
Computerized stationary cycle	Entire lower body
Computerized recumbent cycle	Entire lower body
Computerized upper-body ergometer (UBE)	Entire upper body
Cross-country ski machine	Entire body
Computerized rowing machine	Entire body
Treadmill	Entire body
Climbing machine	Entire body

Miscellaneous Fitness Equipment

Sport cords/elastic therapy bands

Aerobic class step or bench (3 inch–20 inch height)

Stretching mat

Neck pad for Olympic bar

Designing a Home Gym

A home gym obviously needn't have the same equipment as a larger fitness center to meet your basic fitness needs. You should design your home gym based upon the space you have available for equipment and your fitness goals.

The equipment used in a fitness center is usually made for commercial use (heavy use throughout the day). Most manufacturers of commercial fitness equipment also make less expensive versions of their equipment that you can use for your home gym. Manufacturers of home gym equipment usually make a home gym multistation unit for the upper- and lower-body muscle groups. This multistation unit is explained in additional detail later in this chapter.

If possible, you should consult with your own personal fitness trainer before selecting any equipment for your home gym. A fitness professional who knows your specific health history and fitness goals will have a better idea what pieces of equipment will suit your fitness needs.

Home Gym Equipment

Here are some suggestions for selecting single pieces of home gym equipment.

Lower-Body Strength Training Equipment	Focused Muscle Groups Used
Smith press machine for squat exercise and leg press exercise	Entire lower body
Cable column unit	Hips, adductors, abductors, gluteals
Leg extension machine	Quadriceps
Leg curl machine	Hamstrings
6-inch step for calf raises	Calves

Upper-Body Strength Training Equipment	Focused Muscle Groups Used
Smith press machine for chest, shoulder, and upper-back exercises	Entire upper body
Adjustable incline/flat bench	Entire upper body

Flat Olympic bench	Chest, shoulders, triceps
Incline Olympic bench	Chest, shoulders, triceps
Lat pull-down machine	Upper back, biceps, forearms
45-degree back extension	Lower back, hips
Abdominal crunch board	Abdominals, hips, lower back

Free-Weight Equipment for the Upper Body and Lower Body

Olympic bar

E-Z curl bar

Cable bar handles (straight and curved)

Single cable handle

Single cable ankle straps

Free weights plates (2.5 lbs., 5 lbs., 10 lbs., 25 lbs., 35 lbs., 45 lbs.)

Dumbbells (1 lb., 2 lbs., 3 lbs., 5 lbs. 8 lbs., 10 lbs., 12 lbs., 15 lbs., 20 lbs.–50 lbs.)

Cardiovascular Training Equipment (Pick One of the Following)	**Focused Muscle Groups Used**
Stair-climbing machine	Entire lower body
Stationary cycle	Entire lower body
Recumbent cycle	Entire lower body
Computerized stair-climbing machine	Entire lower body

Computerized stationary cycle	Entire lower body
Computerized recumbent cycle	Entire lower body
Computerized upper-body ergometer (UBE)	Entire upper body
Cross-country ski machine	Entire body
Computerized rowing machine	Entire body
Treadmill	Entire body
Climbing machine	Entire body

Miscellaneous Fitness Equipment

Sport cords/elastic therapy bands

Aerobic class step or bench (3 inch–20 inch height)

Stretching mat

Neck pad for Olympic bar

Multistation Units

Multistation units are made for home gym spaces and larger fitness centers; they combine a variety of machines into one machine that you can use to exercise the upper- and lower-body muscle groups. Multistation unit machines usually consist of one to six weight-stacks attached to the following stations:

Lower-Body Strength Training Equipment	**Focused Muscle Groups Used**
Leg press sled	Entire lower body
Squat station	Entire lower body
Cable column unit	Hips, adductors, abductors, gluteals

Leg extension machine	Quadriceps
Leg curl machine	Hamstrings
Standing calf raise machine	Calves

Upper-Body Strength Training Equipment	**Focused Muscle Groups Used**
Assisted dip and chin up machine	Entire upper body
Adjustable incline/flat bench	Entire upper body
Cable column unit	Entire upper body
Chest press machine	Chest, shoulders, triceps
Chest fly machine or peck deck	Chest, shoulders
Incline chest press machine	Chest, shoulders, triceps
Lat pull-down machine	Upper back, biceps, forearms
Abdominal crunch board	Abdominals, hips, lower back

C H A P T E R

3

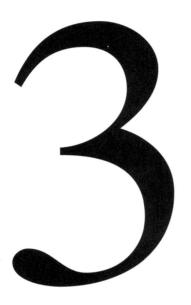

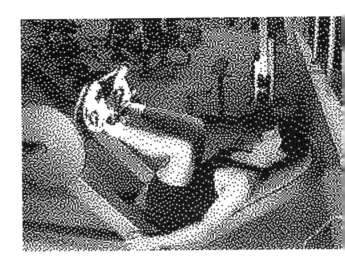

Assessing Your Fitness Level

Personal Fitness Assessment Questionnaire

Fitness Tests

Getting Your Fitness Test Results

Identifying Risk Factors

NO MATTER HOW IN OR OUT OF SHAPE YOU ARE, YOU NEED TO ASSESS your current level of fitness before you can devise a fitness program that is right for you. The personal fitness assessment tests described in this chapter help you determine where you should start. Simply put, they are a series of tests to help you safely and effectively take stock of your current fitness status, enabling you to design a fitness program tailor-made to your individual needs. You can carry out many of these tests at home or at your gym, but in some cases—when determining blood pressure or body fat content, for example—you may need to consult your physician or a trained fitness expert.

You can design your own individual fitness program based on the results of the following six tests:

- Resting state measurements, including blood pressure, heart rate, body weight, and body height

- Body composition measurement to determine your percentage of body fat

- Cardiovascular testing

- Muscular strength testing

- Muscular endurance testing

- Flexibility testing

Personal Fitness Assessment Questionnaire

You should fill out the following questionnaire, which is also found in the "Getting Started" section on the CD-ROM packaged with the book, before participating in any of the personal fitness assessment tests described in this chapter. The questionnaire helps you determine ahead of time whether you have any potential health risks, and, if so, how you should proceed. If there are questions to which you don't know (or are not sure of) the answer, check with your physician or health care provider.

Personal Fitness Assessment Questionnaire

Age _____ Gender _____

Height (in inches) _____ Weight (in pounds) _____

Please indicate if you have a personal history of any of the following conditions. (If you're using the CD-ROM, click on the appropriate answers.)

Heart disease	Yes	No
Abnormal resting EKG	Yes	No

Elevated cholesterol level	Yes	No
Do you smoke cigarettes?	Yes	No
Diabetes mellitus	Yes	No
Obesity	Yes	No
Do you drink alcohol?	Yes	No
Are you over the age of 45?	Yes	No
Are you physically inactive?	Yes	No
Do you have poor nutritional habits?	Yes	No
Do you have a high level of daily stress?	Yes	No
Does your family have a poor medical history?	Yes	No
Gout	Yes	No
Anorexia	Yes	No
Bulimia	Yes	No
Injuries, joint or back pain	Yes	No

If you have answered yes to any of these questions, please refer to the section "Identifying Risk Factors" later in this chapter or to the "Sports Medicine" section on the CD-ROM. If not, it's fine to go directly to the following personal fitness tests, which will help you evaluate your current level of fitness.

Fitness Tests

The personal fitness assessment tests are designed to help you determine your beginning level of fitness, which, in turn, will help you choose the strength training, cardiovascular, and stretching exercises that are right for you. These tests also establish your fitness "baseline." In other words, they serve as markers by which you can calculate your progress when you retake the tests in the future. You should reassess yourself every three months to measure your progress.

To ensure the most accurate results while carrying out your personal fitness assessment, you should follow these guidelines:

1. Make sure to consider any medical or health problems from the past and present. If you are under a physician's care for heart disease, high blood pressure, joint pain, or any other serious health problem, check with your physician or health care provider before performing any of the tests.

2. Avoid any strenuous activity—including any form of exercise—for two hours before taking any of the tests.

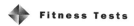

3. Avoid eating a heavy meal right before testing. If you do eat a light meal or snack, you should do so two hours or more before taking any of the tests.

4. Alcohol, caffeine, tobacco, drugs, or any medication may alter your test results, so if possible refrain from using any of these substances 12 hours before you take any of the tests. (If you're on doctor-prescribed medication, keep in mind that your test results may be skewed.)

5. Make sure to wear appropriate athletic attire for the tests. It's best to wear shorts, a short-sleeve T-shirt, and athletic shoes. If you'll be taking the body composition test, avoid leotards and lycra tights because they make it difficult to accurately measure skin folds.

6. When performing any of the personal fitness assessment tests, rest for 3 to 5 minutes between tests to allow for musculoskeletal and cardiovascular recovery.

During some of the tests your blood pressure and heart rate will rise as a result of physical exertion. If you experience dizziness; unusual fatigue or shortness of breath; nausea; chest pain; shooting pain down the left side of your jaw, neck, or arm (heart attack symptoms); or discomfort in your joints, stop exercising immediately. If the symptoms are not life threatening, try to sit down and relax until you feel better.

Resting-state Measurements

You should determine your resting-state measurements for blood pressure, heart rate, body weight, and body height before you take any of the personal fitness assessment tests. If there's not a fitness expert at your gym who can help you with these measurements, please consult your physician or health care provider. You can also have your body fat composition tested by an American College of Sports Medicine–certified health and fitness professional.

Blood Pressure Measurements

You should have your blood pressure measured by an American College of Sports Medicine–certified health and fitness professional or physician before beginning an exercise program with the CD-ROM that accompanies this book.

Blood pressure measurement determines the efficiency of blood flow into and out of the arteries. Actual blood pressure is the force exerted by the blood against the inner walls of the blood vessels, otherwise referred to as *systemic arterial pressure*. Your blood pressure will rise and fall when you exert yourself.

There are two levels of blood pressure measurement. *Systolic blood pressure* is the measurement of blood flow *into* the artery. Systolic blood pressure is known as the active state of blood flow or the maximum pressure achieved when your heart contracts (ventricular contraction). The systolic blood pressure is measured first, and the level of your systolic blood pressure rises when you exercise. The normal range of resting systolic blood pressure should not exceed a level of 140 mm Hg (millimeters of mercury).

Diastolic blood pressure is the measurement of blood flow *out of* the artery. Diastolic blood pressure is known as the resting state of blood flow or the lowest pressure achieved after the ventricular contraction. The diastolic blood pressure is measured second, and the level of your diastolic blood pressure usually stays relatively stable during exercise. The normal range of resting systolic blood pressure should not exceed a level of 90 mm HG (millimeters of mercury).

Resting Heart Rate Measurement

A *resting-state measurement of heart rate* determines the rate at which your heart pumps blood and oxygen into and out of your heart and lungs during a resting state. Heart rates are measured in beats per minute (bpm). Each time your heart contracts (ventricular contraction), there's a heartbeat sound. The American College of Sports Medicine considers a measurement of 60 to 90 heartbeats per minute to be normal, depending upon your age and gender.

You can measure your resting heart rate with your index and middle finger from:

- The radial artery (on the inside of your wrist)

- The carotid artery (under the chin towards the middle of the neck)

- The brachial artery (in between the biceps and triceps muscles on the inside of the arm)

Count your heart rate for 30 seconds and multiply that number by two to determine your beats per minute.

Don't attempt to measure your heart rate with your thumb, since your thumb has a pulse that will disrupt your measurement. If you feel any irregular heart beats while measuring your resting heart rate, please consult your physician before participating in any exercise program.

Body Weight Measurement

To measure your correct body weight, take off your clothes and shoes and stand on a weight scale. You need to know your total body weight mass to determine your level of body fat mass and body mass index. (See the later section "Body Composition Test" for details.)

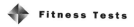

Body Height Measurement

To measure your body height, take off your shoes and stand on a weight/ height scale. Place the ruler on top of your head and stand straight with your back against the scale. If you don't have access to a scale that you can use for height measurements, stand up against the wall (again, with your shoes off) and use a pencil to mark your height on the wall. Then use a tape measure to determine your height. You must know your body height to determine the level of body fat mass and body mass index, as discussed in the next section.

Body Composition Test

The body composition test determines your level of lean body mass percentage versus fat mass percentage (high levels of body fat mass have a direct correlation to coronary artery disease). The body composition measurement is based upon your age, weight, height, and gender.

Before beginning an exercise program, it's a good idea to have a skin fold caliper test performed by an American College of Sports Medicine–certified health and fitness professional to determine your level of body fat mass. This test has a 0 to 3 percent margin of error. All measurements should be taken three times to ensure accuracy. A rest between each measurement permits the fat, blood, and water in your body to return to their original forms before your skin is pinched again.

You may know that men and women carry fat in different places on their body. Men retain the greatest level of body fat in their abdominal area. Women retain the greatest level of body fat in their hips and thighs. For this reason, the skin fold caliper tests for men and women are carried out somewhat differently.

If you're a man, specific measurements are taken at your chest, abdomen, and thigh. The chest measurement is taken on the diagonal fold of the chest, halfway between the nipple and the shoulder joint. The abdominal measurement is taken on the vertical fold of the abdomen, just to the right of the navel. The thigh measurement is taken halfway between the knee cap and the hip crease on the quadriceps.

If you're a woman, specific measurements are taken at your triceps, hip, and thigh. The triceps measurement is taken on the vertical fold of the triceps, halfway between the elbow joint and the shoulder joint. The hip measurement is take on the diagonal fold of the hip, just above the crest of the hip joint. The thigh measurement is taken halfway between the knee cap and the hip crease on the quadriceps.

The American College of Sports Medicine recommends the following levels of body fat for men and women.

	Male	**Female**
Low	6–10% fat	14–18% fat
Optimal	11–17% fat	19–22% fat
Moderate	18–20% fat	23–30% fat
Obesity	Greater than 20% fat	Greater than 30% fat

It's considered unhealthy for men to have a body fat percentage below 3 percent and women to have a body fat percentage below 11 percent. A body fat percentage of over 20 percent for men and over 30 percent for women is also considered unhealthy.

There are a number of body fat misconceptions. One myth is that fat turns to muscle when you exercise. Muscle is a tissue and fat is a substance. Also, muscle weighs approximately 75 percent more than fat; in other words, you can lose fat and gain muscle without losing weight. A second myth is that weighing yourself on a scale is the best way to determine body fat measurement. Feeling how your clothes fit on your body is a much better way to measure body fat loss. You'll also get a better sense of whether you're losing body fat by looking in the mirror with no clothes on.

These three factors affect your body fat level:

- Genetic body type (somatype)

- Daily dietary habits

- Physical activity level

Body Type or Somatype

Somatype is another term for body type. Most people have a genetic predisposition toward one specific somatype and supportive traits from a second somatype. There are three genetic somatypes: ectomorph, mesomorph, and endomorph. An *ectomorph* (endurance athlete) possesses a low body fat percentage level, small bone size, a high metabolism, and a small amount of muscle mass and muscle size. A *mesomorph* (power athlete) possesses a low to medium body fat percentage level, medium to large bone size, a medium to high metabolism, and a large amount of muscle mass and muscle size. An *endomorph* (nonathlete) possesses a high body fat percentage level, large bone size, a slow metabolism, and a small amount of muscle mass and muscle size.

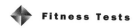

Your body type is something you're born with and can't necessarily change. However, you obviously *can* change your dietary habits and level of physical activity to positively affect your body fat percentage and fitness level.

Dietary Habits

What you eat and the way you eat can greatly affect your body fat level as well as your overall health and well-being. Your nutritional needs will obviously vary depending upon your health and fitness goals. At the same time, even if your health goals are modest, it's a good idea to get some sense of nutition's role in total fitness. You may be pleasantly surprised to find that you can make minor changes to your eating habits and end up with a much healthier diet. Chapter 6 and the "Nutrition" section on the CD-ROM cover the topic of nutrition in more detail, but if you want specific dietary recommendations, you should consult your doctor or a registered dietitian.

Physical Activity Level

The amount of exercise you get has a profound effect upon your level of body fat. If you increase your physical activity level, you will expend greater amounts of calories and fat, depending on how long and at what level of intensity you exercise. Here are some general guidelines:

- Consistent aerobic/cardiovascular exercise (20 minutes, three times per week) will improve your cardiovascular system, increase your metabolism, and burn body fat. For additional details on cardiovascular training routines that will suit your needs, consult Chapter 5 and the "Personal Fitness Training Program" section on the CD-ROM.

- Consistent weight/strength training (20 minutes, three times per week) will increase your muscular strength, enhance your muscular endurance, result in a leaner body mass, and favorably affect your bone density. For in-depth coverage of strength training routines, refer to the "Personal Fitness Training Program" section on the CD-ROM.

- Stretching before and after exercise will increase the range of motion of your joints and muscles. Increasing your flexibility also decreases your risk of injury while exercising. For descriptions of various stretching exercises, refer to the "Personal Fitness Training Program" section on the CD-ROM.

Submaximal Cardiovascular (VO2) Capacity Test

The submaximal cardiovascular test determines the amount of oxygen that you will consume and expend during aerobic exercise. The VO2 capacity test (volume of oxygen test) lets you determine the safest and most efficient target heart rate range and oxygen level during cardiovascular exercise.

The American College of Sports Medicine recommends that you maintain a 50- to 90-percent level of your age-predicted maximal heart rate intensity during aerobic activity. A level of 85 percent is the termination point of the submaximal test. If you're at an advanced level of fitness, you can aim for a 90 percent level of age-predicted maximal heart rate. In a moment, you'll learn how to determine your age-predicted maximal heart rate.

If your blood pressure exceeds 220 over 110—that is, a reading of over 220 systolic blood pressure and over 110 diastolic blood pressure—during the cardiovascular test described shortly, you should stop the test.

How to Determine a Safe Target Heart Rate Zone

A critical part of your cardiovascular (VO2) test is to determine a safe and effective target rate zone for aerobic exercise. Setting a specific target heart rate zone helps you determine when you have reached your submaximal level heart rate of 85 percent.

As you learned earlier in the chapter, you should measure your heart rate by placing the index and middle finger—not the thumb—on the carotid artery, radial artery, or brachial artery. Remember, your heart rate (HR) is measured in beats per minute (bpm).

Age-Predicted Maximal Heart Rate

220 – age _____ = Max HR _____ bpm

Max HR × 50% = _____ bpm

Max HR × 90% = _____ bpm

Optimum Training HR Zone (50%–90%)   = _____ bpm

= _____ bpm/10 sec

In other words, if you're 35, your age-predicted maximal heart rate is 185 beats per minute (220–35), 50 percent of your maximal heart rate is 92.5 beats per minute (185 × 50%), and 90 percent of your maximal heart rate is 166.5 beats per minute (185 × 90%). That is, your optimum training heart rate zone is between 92.5 and 166.5 beats per minute, or between approximately 15 and 27 beats every 10 seconds.

If you use the Karvonen system instead, you first need to measure your heart rate. (Your Karvonen training heart rate level indicates the most effective aerobic training heart rate range for cardiovascular exercise.)

Karvonen Training Heart Rate Method

220 – age _____ = Max HR _____ bpm

Max HR _____ – Resting HR _____ = Functional HR _____

Functional HR × 60% + Resting HR = Training HR _____ bpm

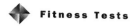
Functional HR × 80% + Resting HR = Training HR _____ bpm

Optimum Training HR Zone (60%–80%) = _____ bpm

= _____ bpm/10 sec

As an example, if you're 35 and your resting heart rate is 65 beats per minute, your "functional heart rate" would be 120. (220 minus 35 is 185, and 185 minus 65 is 120.) Then you take 60 percent of your functional heart rate and add it to your resting heart rate for the low measurement, and you take 80 percent of your functional heart rate and add it to your resting heart rate for the high measurement. According to these calculations, the optimum training heart rate zone for the person in this example would be between 137 and 161, or between approximately 22 and 26 beats every 10 seconds.

YMCA Step Test

You can use the YMCA step test to determine a baseline measurement for your cardiovascular capacity. To get an accurate measurement, you should use a 12-inch step or bench for the test. It's best if you have a metronome to measure beats per minute while stepping.

1. Begin by stepping up and down on the 12-inch step or bench at 96 beats per minute for three consecutive minutes.

2. Measure your heart rate and enter the number into the worksheet of the CD-ROM accompanying this book. You'll receive a measurement of fitness level and V02 maximum.

Because the YMCA step test is a beginning level test, the results may be somewhat skewed for exercisers at intermediate or advanced levels of fitness. If you fall into either of these categories, you should have your V02 Max measured using a graded exercise test with a treadmill (the Naughton-Balke test) or cycle ergometer (the Astrand-Rhyming test) by an American College of Sports Medicine–certified health and fitness professional or physician before beginning an exercise program with the CD-ROM. These more strenuous tests will more accurately determine your level of oxygen capacity.

After completing the VO2 test, allow yourself to recover for 3 to 5 minutes before beginning your muscular strength and muscular endurance tests.

Muscular Strength and Endurance Tests

The muscular strength test determines the maximal amount of weight that you can lift with your upper body, measuring the muscular strength of your chest, shoulders, and triceps. *Muscular strength* is the measurement of increases in overall strength and speed in the muscle during a movement. Exercises that build up your muscular strength involve lifting increasingly heavy volumes of weight with minimal repetitions to produce maximum power within the muscles being used.

An example of a muscular strength exercise is to lift 120 pounds for ten repetitions during the first set of barbell chest presses, and then to lift 150 pounds for seven repetitions during the second set of barbell chest presses.

The YMCA Bench Press Test

The YMCA bench press test involves lifting a weighted barbell with your upper body for as many repetitions as you can at a 60 beat per minute count. Men should use an 80-pound barbell and women should use a 35-pound barbell for the test. If you cannot lift these recommended weights, do the push-up test instead. You should use a metronome for this test if you can.

You should only perform this test if you're at an intermediate or advanced fitness level. In addition, you shouldn't carry out the test without the presence of another person for proper spotting and safety.

1. Begin the bench press test by lifting the weighted barbell off the barbell rack and holding the barbell directly above the midline of the chest (nipple line).

2. Keep a 60 beat per minute cadence with the metronome during this test. While you are performing this test, the barbell should either be touching your chest or fully extended during each beat of the metronome.

3. Once you break the cadence or can no longer lift the barbell, the test is terminated.

4. After you complete this bench press test, record the number of repetitions into the CD-ROM worksheet. You will receive a correlated measurement of fitness level.

Refer to the "Personal Fitness Training Program" section on the CD-ROM for further information about muscular strength and determining weight volume for strength training exercises. After completing the YMCA bench press test, make sure to take 3 to 5 minutes to recover before performing any other personal fitness assessment tests.

The Maximal Bench Press Test

The maximal bench press test involves lifting one time the maximal amount of weight on a barbell with your upper body. A full repetition is recorded if you can elevate the barbell from the midline (nipple line) of your chest upwards until your arms are fully extended. If you cannot extend your arms fully, the lift does not count. *You should only perform this test if you're at an intermediate or advanced fitness level.* This test is not included on the CD-ROM.

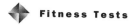
1. Begin the test by using a weighted barbell that is equal to 50 percent of your body weight, for men, or 30 percent, for women. You should lift this barbell 10 to 15 times to warm up your upper-body muscles.

2. After the warm-up set, take a 90-second rest before beginning the first one-repetition maximal bench press.

3. Increase the weight volume on the barbell by 10 percent and perform a one-repetition bench press. Then take another 90-second rest period before the next lift.

4. Keep repeating step 3 until you reach a weight that you can no longer lift.

5. After you have lifted the heaviest weight possible for one full repetition, record the amount lifted as the "maximal weight." If you can lift 135 percent of your body weight one time, you have good upper-body strength.

After completing the maximal bench press test, take 3 to 5 minutes to recover before beginning the muscular endurance tests.

Muscular Endurance Tests

The tests covered here measure the muscular endurance of your upper body and mid-torso. Muscular endurance is the muscle's ability to withstand isolated or overall effects of fatigue on the body during a movement. Exercises that build up your muscular endurance involve lifting light to moderate volumes of weight with maximal repetitions to produce maximal endurance within the muscles being used.

 An example of a muscular endurance exercise is to increase the number of times (repetitions) that a muscle contracts while you lift 120 pounds of weight during a barbell chest press. Refer to the "Personal Fitness Training Program" section on the CD-ROM for more information about muscular endurance.

Abdominal Crunch Test

The one-minute abdominal crunch test measures the muscular endurance of your abdominal wall muscles. You count the total number of repetitions that you can perform in 1 minute straight.

1. Position yourself on your back on the floor with your knees bent and your heels 12 to 18 inches from your buttocks.

2. Place your hands behind your head or crossed against your chest and lift your upper torso towards the ceiling so that your shoulders elevate one to three inches off of the ground; then return your upper torso to the ground. Alternatively, place your hands along the sides of your body and move your hands three inches forward each time you lift the upper torso.

3. Repeat step 2 for a full minute. Note that a repetition is only counted if you elevate your shoulder blades one to three inches off the ground or if your hands move three inches forward during the test. A repetition is also not counted if you lift your feet or lower back off the ground. Make sure not to use your hips for momentum.

4. Enter the maximum number of repetitions you completed in one minute into the CD-ROM worksheet. You will receive a correlated measurement of fitness level.

After completing the test, give yourself 3 to 5 minutes of rest before going on to the next test.

Push-Up Test

The push-up test measures the muscular endurance of your upper body. (This test is optional and is not included on the CD-ROM.) This test has no time limit. Perform as many push-ups as you can without stopping to rest.

1. Position yourself face down on the floor, place your hands a little wider than shoulder width, and keep a straight back—this is a military style push-up. Men should perform the push-up with their knees off the ground. Women should perform the push-up with their knees on the ground.

2. Keeping your back straight, straighten your arms completely, raising your body up off the floor. Then bend your arms and lower your body until it's almost touching the floor.

3. Repeat step 2 until you have to stop to rest or can no longer perform a full push-up. You must keep your back straight throughout the test. If your back bends, the test is terminated. Also, you cannot stop to rest in a locked arm position. Once you cannot move in full continuation of the movement, the test is terminated.

4. Record the maximum amount of repetitions you completed. If you can perform 20 or more push-ups, you have good upper-body muscular endurance.

After completing the push-up test, rest for 3 to 5 minutes before taking any further tests.

Flexibility Test

An increase in pelvic tilt may occur if you have tight hamstring muscles and iliopsoas (hip) muscles. This may have an adverse effect on the flexibility of your lower back. It is important to increase your flexibility to avoid injury and to elongate the muscle groups. Greater muscle length helps to produce greater muscle size and muscle strength.

Sit-and-Reach Flexibility Test

The sit-and-reach test determines the flexibility of your trunk, lower back, pelvic girdle, and hamstrings. *This test may cause pain and injuries to the hamstrings, spine, and lower back.* If you have any prior injuries in these areas, do not perform the test.

1. Sit on the floor with your legs extended under a sit-and-reach box or place a tape measure underneath your legs. Your heels should be on the floor and your toes should extend straight up.

2. Place your hands on top of one another and reach forward with your hands together, bending at the hips without bending the knees. If you're using the sit-and-reach box, push the block forward. If you're using the tape measure, place the 14-inch tape measurement mark at the base of your heels and extend the tape measure forward. Measure the line from the top of your fingers to the tape measurement below.

3. Exhale while extending your upper torso forward during the sit-and-reach test.

4. Measure your extended reach three times and take the average of all three reaches as your total, which you should enter into the CD-ROM worksheet. You'll receive a correlated measurement of fitness level.

   Please refer to Chapter 5 and the "Personal Fitness Training Program" section on the CD-ROM for further information about stretching and flexibility.

Getting Your Fitness Test Results

After you complete the personal fitness assessment tests and enter the results in the CD-ROM worksheet, press the Score button to get an accurate assessment of your fitness level. You can print a test result sheet at this time. Once you determine your fitness level—beginning, intermediate, or advanced—the next step is to design and implement your individual fitness program by selecting the proper strength training, cardiovascular training, and flexibility exercises from the "Personal Fitness Training Program" section on the CD-ROM. Chapter 5 also has information on designing your personal fitness program.

Identifying Risk Factors

This section will help you identify the primary, secondary, and possible risk factors associated with overall health according to the American College of Sports Medicine. Understanding these risk factors can help you determine what level of fitness program is appropriate for you. If you have three or more of the primary or secondary risk factors, or you have two primary risk factors and one or more secondary risk factors, consult your physician before beginning an exercise program.

Primary Risk Factors

There are five primary risk factors: smoking, hypertension (high blood pressure), hyperlipidemia (elevated cholesterol), diabetes mellitus (blood glucose), and abnormal resting EKG (electrocardiogram).

Smoking
Smoking is the number one risk factor for causing coronary heart disease, cancer, and other major health risks. The fewer cigarettes you smoke in a day, the lower your risk of coronary artery disease. The levels of risk are as follows:

Low Risk	Less than 10 cigarettes per day
Moderate Risk	10 to 19 cigarettes per day
High Risk	20 or more cigarettes per day

Hypertension (High Blood Pressure)
Hypertension is one of the leading causes of heart attacks, strokes, and other heart-related diseases. The recommended levels of blood pressure are as follows:

Optimal	Less than 145/95 mm Hg
Moderate Risk	145-159/95 mm Hg
High Risk	160/95 mm Hg

Incorporating some type of fitness program into your lifestyle and moderating your level of fatty food intake may help decrease your blood pressure.

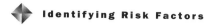

Hyperlipidemia (Elevated Cholesterol)

A high cholesterol level is another leading cause of heart attacks, strokes, and other heart-related diseases. The recommended cholesterol levels are as follows:

Total Cholesterol

Optimal	Less than 200 mg/dl
Moderate Risk	200–239 mg/dl
High	Greater than 240 mg/dl

Total Cholesterol/High Density Lipoprotein (TC/HDL)

Optimal	3.2–3.9
Moderate Risk	4–5
High Risk	Greater than 5

Triglycerides (Trans Fatty Acids)

Optimal	Less than 100 mg/dl
Moderate Risk	100–249 mg/dl
High Risk	Greater than 250 mg/dl

You should get your cholesterol levels tested by your physician, who should be able to give you a complete description of your cholesterol ratios, what they mean, and possible dietary measures or medications for altering moderate or high-risk cholesterol levels.

Diabetes Mellitus (Blood Glucose)

High blood sugar levels increase your risk for diabetes mellitus, which is the number one cause of blindness. Before beginning an exercise program, you should have your physician or health care provider check your blood sugar level. The recommended levels of blood sugar per day are as follows:

Optimal	Less than 115 mg/dl
Moderate Risk	115–179 mg/dl
High Risk	Greater than 180 mg/dl

Abnormal Resting EKG (Electrocardiogram)

An abnormal resting EKG is an indicator of coronary disease. Check with your physican or health care provider before embarking on an exercise program. The recommended levels are as follows:

Optimal	No abnormalities
Moderate Risk	Bundle branch block
	a. ST segment changes
	b. Ventricular arrhythmias
	c. Abnormal t-waves
	d. Left ventricle strain patterns
High Risk	Acute myocardial infarction (heart attack)
	a. Left ventricular hypertrophy
	b. Ischemia
	c. Conduction defects
	d. Dysrhythmias

Secondary Risk Factors

There are six secondary risk factors: age and gender, physical inactivity, obesity, poor daily nutritional habits, high stress levels, and heredity.

Age and Gender

Age and gender can have a significant role in any health risk. The older you are, the greater your risk of coronary heart disease. If you're a male over the age of 45 years or a female over the age of 50 years, you're at an increased risk for heart attack and other heart-related diseases. If you fall into either of these categories, you should check with your physician or health care provider before beginning a fitness program.

Physical Inactivity

Physical inactivity increases your risk for coronary heart disease. The recommended levels of caloric expenditure are as follows:

Optimal	5,000 Kcals per week
Moderate Risk	500–5,000 Kcals per week
High Risk	Fewer than 500 Kcals per week

Caloric expenditure depends upon numerous factors, including your age, weight, height, and body fat percentage. Again, check with your physician or health care provider to help you determine what amount of physical activity you'll need to perform to fall within safe and healthy levels of caloric expenditure.

Obesity

Obesity increases your risk for coronary heart disease. See the section "Body Composition Test" earlier in this chapter for details on the recommended levels of body fat for men and women, information about what factors affect body fat percentages, and more.

Poor Daily Nutritional Habits

A poor diet will increase your risk of coronary heart disease and leave you vulnerable to nutritional deficiencies that can affect your daily life. The recommended dietary breakdown levels for a healthy daily diet are

- 30% fat
- 50% carbohydrates
- 20% protein

As you may know, foods that are high in fat include red meat, nuts, cheese, ice cream, cooking oils, and avocados. Foods that are high in carbohydrates include breads, pasta, and potatoes. Foods that are high in protein include egg whites, chicken (white meat), beans, and skim milk. For additional details on nutrition and fitness, refer to Chapter 6. For specific diet recommendatins, consult your doctor or a registered dietitian

High Stress Levels

High levels of mental stress have been linked to cancer, heart disease, and high blood pressure. A lower level of daily stress will decrease most adverse health risks. Incidentally, an excellent way of lowering your stress level is to exercise.

Heredity

If your family has a history of heart disease or other health problems, you're at an increased risk for adverse health risks. The levels of risk are as follows:

Optimal	No family history
Moderate Risk	Old myocardial infarction (heart attack), angina, or stroke in siblings or parents aged 50 or more years.
High Risk	Old myocardial infarction (heart attack), angina, or stroke in siblings or parents aged less than 50 years.

Possible Risk Factors

There are three possible risk factors: gout, alcohol consumption, and anorexia and bulimia.

Gout

Gout is caused by high levels of uric acid content in the blood. Gout leads to major problems in the joints of the body and blood stream. The recommended uric acid levels are as follows:

Low Risk	Less than 6.5 uric acid
Moderate Risk	6.5–8.5 uric acid
Health Risk	Greater than 8.5 uric acid

Alcohol Consumption

Alcohol consumption may increase your chances of cancer, heart disease, liver deterioration, and muscle stimulus impediment. The amount of alcohol that can be considered a safe consumption level (as relates to overall health and fitness) differs widely among individuals. Factors such as family medical history, the presence of heart disease, and medications all play a part in determining how much alcohol a person can consume and remain healthy. As a very general rule of thumb, the maximum amount of alcohol a person can consume and still remain healthy is no more than two drinks per day. One drink is defined as 1 ounce of hard alcohol, 3 ounces of wine, or 12 ounces of beer. If you have questions about how much alcohol is too much for you, consult your physician.

Anorexia and Bulimia

A history of anorexia (not eating) or bulimia (eating and regurgitating the food afterwards) can increase your risk of bone density loss, muscle tissue loss, and even death from starvation. The recommended level of body mass index is as follows:

Health Risk   Body mass index less than 1

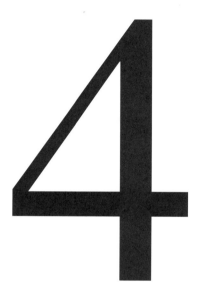

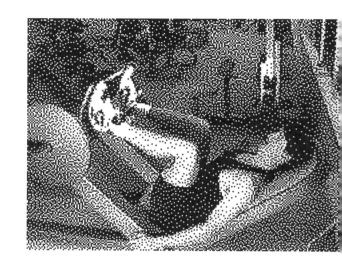

Muscular and Skeletal Anatomy: A Crash Course

Muscular Anatomy
Skeletal Anatomy
Planes of the Body
Kinesiology/Physiology

BEFORE YOU BEGIN AN EXERCISE PROGRAM, IT'S A GOOD IDEA TO educate yourself a bit about human anatomy. If you understand how your body operates when you exercise, you have a better idea of how to avoid injuries. You may also gain a clearer idea of where you want to go, in terms of fitness, and the best way to get there. Learning about anatomy can provide you with an inside picture of what's happening when you carry out your fitness program.

Muscular Anatomy

This section focuses on the human muscular system (see Figure 4.1). Table 4.1 lists the major muscle groups. The muscle groups are divided into smaller muscle groups, each of which has its own particular function within the skeletal system.

Table 4.1   **Muscle Groups in the Human Body**

Lower Body Muscle Groups

Major Muscle Groups	Muscle Subgroups
Gluteal muscles (buttocks)	Gluteus maximus Gluteus medius
Quadriceps muscles (thighs**)**	Vastus medialus Vastus lateralis Vastus intermedius Rectus femoris Sartorius
Hamstrings muscles (rear upper leg)	Biceps femoris Semimembranosus Semitendinosus
Abductor muscles (outer thigh)	Tensor faciae latae
Adductor muscles	Pectineous
Calf muscles (lower leg)	Soleus Gastocnemius Anterior tibialis Posterior tibialis Flexor digitorum longus Extensor digitorum longus Peroneus longus Peroneus tertias Peroneus brevis Extensor hallucis tongus

Continued on page 42

Figure 4.1

The human muscular system

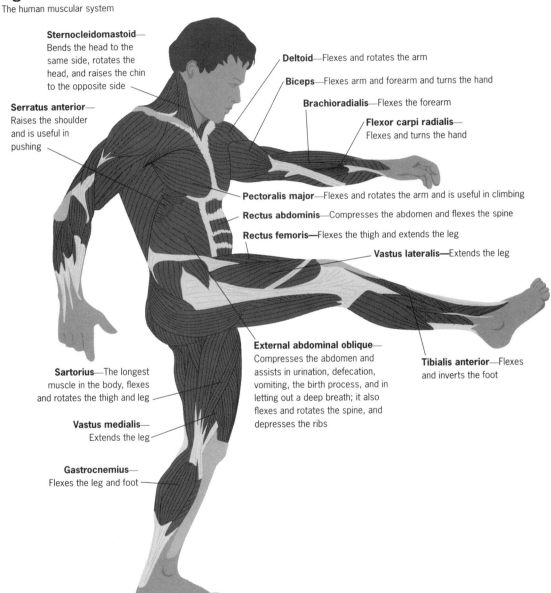

Sternocleidomastoid—Bends the head to the same side, rotates the head, and raises the chin to the opposite side

Serratus anterior—Raises the shoulder and is useful in pushing

Deltoid—Flexes and rotates the arm

Biceps—Flexes arm and forearm and turns the hand

Brachioradialis—Flexes the forearm

Flexor carpi radialis—Flexes and turns the hand

Pectoralis major—Flexes and rotates the arm and is useful in climbing

Rectus abdominis—Compresses the abdomen and flexes the spine

Rectus femoris—Flexes the thigh and extends the leg

Vastus lateralis—Extends the leg

Sartorius—The longest muscle in the body, flexes and rotates the thigh and leg

Vastus medialis—Extends the leg

Gastrocnemius—Flexes the leg and foot

External abdominal oblique—Compresses the abdomen and assists in urination, defecation, vomiting, the birth process, and in letting out a deep breath; it also flexes and rotates the spine, and depresses the ribs

Tibialis anterior—Flexes and inverts the foot

Trapezius—Raises, turns, and lowers the shoulder and turns the face to the same or the opposite side

Teres major—Extends and rotates the arm

Triceps—Extends and rotates the arm and extends the forearm

Extensor carpi radialis longus—Extends and turns the hand

Infraspinatus—Rotates the arm

Extensor carpi ulnaris—Extends and turns the hand

Deltoid—Flexes and rotates the arm

Flexor carpi ulnaris—Flexes and turns the hand

Latissmus dorsi—Extends and rotates the arm, draws the shoulder down and back, and helps in climbing

External abdominal oblique

Gluteus medius—Turns, rotates, and can also flex or extend the thigh

Semitendinosus—Extends the thigh and flexes the leg. After it is flexed, can rotate it

Gluteus maximus—Extends and rotates the thigh and braces the knee

Biceps femoris—Extends the thigh and rotates it, and flexes the leg and rotates it

Semimembranosus—Flexes the leg, and after it is flexed, may rotate it. Also extends the thigh

Gastrocnemius—Forms the bulk of the calf of the leg and flexes the leg and foot

Soleus—Flexes the foot

Table 4.1   Muscle Groups in the Human Body (Continued)

Adductor muscles (inner thigh)	Adductor longus
	Adductor magnus
	Brevis
	Gracilis

Upper Body Muscle Groups

Major Muscle Groups	Muscle Subgroups
Chest muscles	Pectoralis major
	Pectoralis minor
Upper back muscles	Latissimus dorsi
	Rhomboids
	Subscapularis
	Serratus anterior
	Teres major
	Teres minor
Anterior hip muscles	Psoas major (flexor)
	Psoas minor (flexor)
	Sartorius (flexor)
Lower back muscles	Erector spinae
	Quadratus lumborum (posterior hip extensor)
Shoulder muscles	Anterior deltoid (front)
	Medial/lateral deltoid (middle)
	Posterior deltoid (rear)
	Trapezius
Rotator cuff muscles (inner shoulder)	Supraspinatus
	Infraspinatus
	Teres major
	Subscapularis
Triceps muscles (posterior upper arm)	Triceps brachii (lateral long head)
	Triceps brachii (medial long head)
	Triceps brachii (medial short head)
	Brachioradialis
Biceps muscles (anterior upper arm)	Brachialis (lower head)
	Biceps brachii (upper heads)
	Brachioradialis

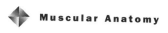
Table 4.1	Muscle Groups in the Human Body (Continued)	
Forearm muscles (lower arm)		Pronator teres
		Brachioradialis
		Supinator
		Extensor carpi radialis longus
		Extensor carpi radialis brevis
Abdominal muscles (mid torso)		External obliques (outside)
		Internal oblique (outside)
		Rectus abdominis (upper)
		Transverse abdominis (lower)

Muscles

Muscle is a connective tissue that supports the skeletal system. Muscles can shorten and lengthen continuously without too much complication.

Muscle fibers are comprised of extrafusal fibers and intrafusal fibers. Extrafusal fibers are made up of filaments called myofibrils, which in turn are comprised of several interconnected bands. These myofibrils can relax, contract, and lengthen the muscle. In between these myofibril bands are sarcomeres. Inside the sarcomere are protein myofilaments known as actin (thin filament) and myosin (thick filament). The myosin creates small projectiles called cross bridges. The cross bridges are stimulated by a chemical reaction (acetylcholine release) in the brain that causes the actin and myosin to slide over one another, allowing the muscle to shorten and lengthen.

Intrafusal fibers are muscle spindles that act as the stretch receptors in the muscle. The stretch receptor reflex receives neurological messages from the brain.

When the extrafusal fibers and intrafusal fibers interact with one another, the brain's messages make the muscle shorten and lengthen. This is known as muscle contraction.

Three Types of Muscle Fibers

The human body includes three types of muscle fibers: fast glycotic muscle, slow oxidative muscle, and fast oxidative glycotic muscle.

Slow oxidative muscles, or SO muscles, are comprised of red muscle fibers. These types of muscles produce greater oxygen levels within the muscle. They include a high concentration of mitochondria cells—the main energy producing cell of the human body. This cell creates greater levels of oxygen capacity for the muscle. Most endurance athletes possess a high quantity of slow oxidative muscle fiber in their genetic physiology.

Fast glycotic muscles, or FG muscles, are comprised of white muscle fibers. These types of muscles facilitate muscular strength (power and speed) during an exercise movement. They are more compact (dense) than the other types of muscle fibers. Most strength athletes possess a high ratio of fast glycotic muscle fiber in their genetic physiology.

Fast oxidative glycotic muscles, or FOG muscles, are comprised of white muscle fibers and red muscle fibers. These types of muscles produce equal distribution of oxygen and strength within the muscle. Many elite athletes have a high quantity of fast oxidative glycotic muscle fiber in their genetic physiology.

Tendons and Ligaments

Aside from muscles, two other anatomical connective tissues provide support and mobility to the musculoskeletal system:

- Tendons connect muscles to bone.

- Ligaments connect bone to bone.

Both tendons and ligaments (see Figure 4.2) can lengthen or shorten, but you risk injury if you stretch either too far.

Figure 4.2
Tendons and ligaments are also connective tissue.

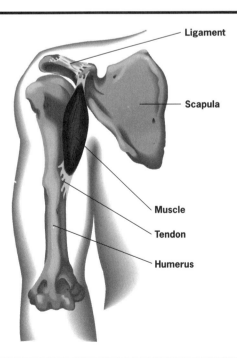

Ligament

Scapula

Muscle

Tendon

Humerus

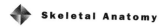
Skeletal Anatomy

This section will help you understand the skeletal system (see Figure 4.3) and how it works in conjunction with the muscular system.

Your skeletal system has three primary functions:

■ It support your muscular system.

■ It protects your nervous system and inner organs.

■ It permits you to move your muscular system. In this sense, it is referred to as your lever system.

The skeletal system refers to the bones of the human body as well as the joints that are attached to those bones. Two types of tissue make up the skeletal system: bone tissue and cartilage tissue.

Bones

Bones are made up of tissue that consists of both living and nonliving cells. The nonliving cells (intracellular) are calcified. Calcification makes the bones rigid, helping them to support the muscular system. The living cells help the bones to regenerate themselves if there is a break or contusion.

Bones consist of several components (see Figure 4.4):

■ The diaphysis is the shaft of the bone. Its main function is to provide support.

■ The epiphysis is the end of each bone. It is referred to as the extremity of the bone and helps maintain the stability of the joint and bone interaction.

■ The medullary cavity is inside the bone shaft and is filled with bone marrow. The bone marrow runs along the length of the bone shaft.

■ The endosteum is a membrane that lines the medullary cavity.

■ Periosteum is a fibrous membrane that protects the bones. The periosteum interlaces with muscle tendons to anchor the bone to the muscle.

Types of Bones

The skeletal system includes four types of bones:

■ Long bones are comprised of all six bone components—the diaphysis, epiphysis, medullary cavity, endosteum, periosteum, and articular cartilage.

■ Short bones are comprised of cancellous bone (spongy/porous bone) that is between one layer of compact bone.

Figure 4.3

The human skeletal system

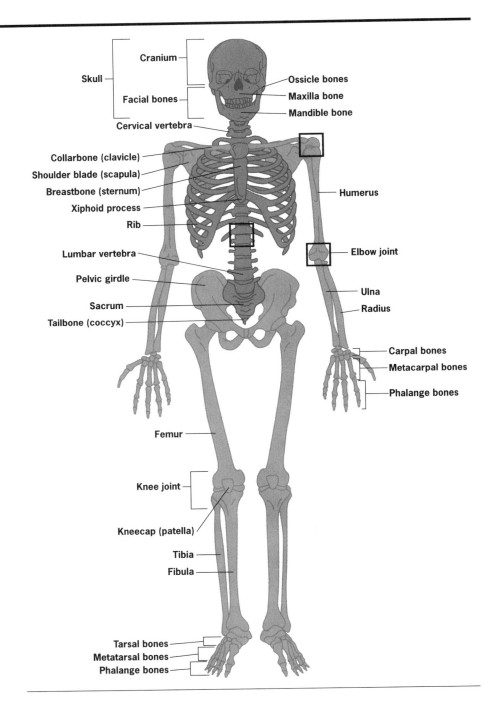

Figure 4.4
The structure of
bone

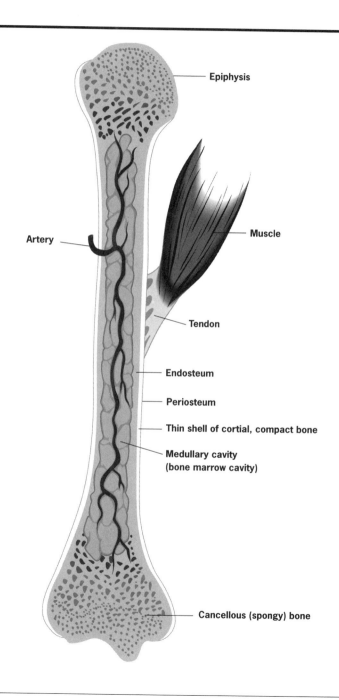

Epiphysis

Artery

Muscle

Tendon

Endosteum

Periosteum

Thin shell of cortial, compact bone

Medullary cavity
(bone marrow cavity)

Cancellous (spongy) bone

- Flat bones are made up of cancellous bone that are between two layers of compact bone.

- Irregular bones consist of cancellous bone that are between one layer of compact bone.

Table 4.2 lists examples of the four bone types.

Table 4.2   **Bone Types and Examples**

Bone Type	Bones in the Skeletal System
Long bones	Femur, tibia, fibula, humerus, radius, ulna, clavicle, phalanges
Short bones	Carpals, tarsals
Flat bones	Ribs, sternum, scapula, patella, cranial
Irregular bones	Pelvic girdle, vertebrae, coccyx, sacrum, hyoid

---

Articular Cartilage

Between each bone and joint is a pillowy tissue called cartilage, which cushions the bones. The articular cartilage outlines the epiphysis of each end of the bone. The cartilage provides a buffer for bones to move against each other within the joint.

Planes of the Body

The planes of the body divide the anatomy into four subsections. The body's specific center of gravity is defined by the intersection of these four planes: sagital, mid-sagital, coronal, and transverse.

The sagital plane extends from the front of the body to the back of the body, or anterior-posterior plane. The mid-sagital plane divides the body into two halves, right-left halves. The coronal plane extends through the middle of the body from one side of the body to the other side, it divides the body into two halves, the front and back. The transverse plane extends through the middle of the body dividing the lower half of the body and the upper half of the body.

Kinesiology/Physiology

Kinesiology is the study of muscle movement. Muscle movement occurs when there is any type of physiological stress upon the muscles during a particular exercise or action. This section should help you understand the concept of kinesiology and the different musculoskeletal movements of the human anatomy.

Muscle Contractions

A muscle contraction is any accelerated, decelerated, or static movement that occurs during an exercise or activity.

A concentric contraction is the positive movement of the exercise. During the concentric contraction, the muscle is shortened and the exercise motion is the ascending action (pushing and pulling). An example of a concentric contraction is the shortening of the biceps brachii during the upward curling motion of the unilateral cable biceps curl exercise.

An eccentric contraction is the negative movement of the exercise. During the eccentric contraction, the muscle is lengthened and the exercise motion is the descending action (releasing and lowering). An example of an eccentric contraction is the lengthening of the biceps brachii during the downward motion of the barbell biceps curl exercise.

An isometric contraction is a static movement exercise. During the isometric contraction, the muscle is neither shortened or lengthened. An example of a isometric contraction is the static movement of the quadriceps muscles group during an isometric wall sit exercise.

Physiological Responses to Muscle Contractions

The body's physiological response to exercise involves adaptations to stress put upon the muscle. As the stress intensifies, the muscle cells produce increased energy storage, transportation, and utilization.

Muscle cells need to continuously respond to greater stimulus each time you increase the stress upon the muscle. This overload factor increases the efficiency of the energy stored within the muscle cell.

The body receives energy from the different types of calories we eat (proteins, fats, and carbohydrates). For further details about calories and nutrition, refer to Chapter 6 or the "Nutrition" section on the CD-ROM.

The initial energy source for muscle contraction is from fat and carbohydrate calories that break down chemically to become stored energy in the body:

■ Adenosine triphosphate (ATP) is a complex chemical compound that is formed from energy released by foods digested by the body. ATP is stored in the muscle cells of the body.

- Creatine phosphate (CP) is a chemical compound stored in the muscle cell; it breaks down to manufacture ATP.

- Myoglobin is an oxygen binding substance that stores and diffuses oxygen, and gives red muscle fibers its color.

Energy sources supplied to the body are dependent upon intensity and time of the muscle's activity.

Short-term energy (ATP-CP energy) is a chemically stored energy source in the body that supplies energy to the muscle for approximately 30 seconds in length. Any intense muscle contraction that happens for longer than 5–10 seconds requires continuous ATP replenishment. As the ATP-CP energy source decreases, the muscle will begin to fatigue.

Prolonged-term energy is an energy source created from carbohydrates (muscle and liver glycogen) and fat (muscle triglcyerides), combined with blood substrates that include lactic acid (a substance produced by a metabolic reaction resulting from the incomplete breakdown of stored glucose). Free fatty acids and glucose help to produce ATP replenishment.

Glycolytic/lactic acid system is an energy source produced anaerobically (without oxygen) by the breakdown of muscle glycogen (stored sugar in the muscle) and pyruvic acid (the substance formed by the incomplete chemical breakdown of glycogen, which occurs during aerobic glycolosis only). This breakdown is the precursor to the build up of the lactic acid system (the anaerobic energy system that occurs when glucose breakdown is incomplete forming lactic acid within the muscle). This energy source occurs in intense muscle contractions lasting 30–120 seconds in length.

The anaerobic/aerobic energy system is an energy source that is the combination of the aerobic system (the energy system that replenishes ATP and pyruvic acid rapidly) and the anaerobic system (the energy system that produces lactic acid system). In this energy system, fats can enter the aerobic pathway and glycogen metabolizes in the lactic acid pathway. This energy system occurs in intense muscle contractions lasting 3–5 minutes in length.

The oxidative energy system is produced by the replenishment of glycogen, which produces pyruvic acid and creates a greater amount of aerobic energy capacity. During an increase in aerobic energy capacity there is an increase in myoglobin storage and aerobic enzymes (proteins compounds that speed the chemical reaction process that facilitates oxygen storage and diffusion). Another increase occurs in the volume and density of mitochondria (a subcellular structure found in all aerobic cells of the muscle). Mitochondria produce the greatest amount of aerobic energy in the muscle. This energy system occurs in intense muscle contractions that last longer than 5 minutes.

Skeletal Joint Movements

This section explains the variety of skeletal joint movements (see Figure 4.5). A muscle's movement directly correlates to the ranges of motion a joint may move through during an exercise movement or activity.

Figure 4.5

The human body has three types of joints: the ball and socket (a), as in the shoulder joint; the hinge (b), as in the elbow; and a gliding joint (c), as in the spine's bones and vertebrae.

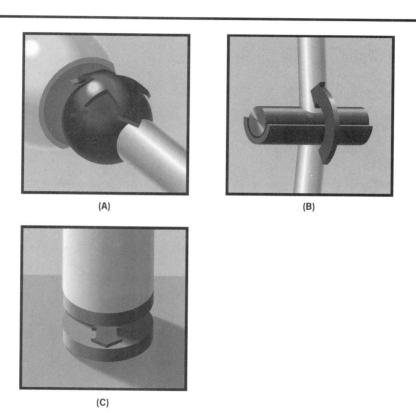

(A)

(B)

(C)

Range of motion refers to the entire movement of the musculoskeletal system during an exercise movement. You should emphasize a slow and controlled movement throughout the full range of motion of an exercise to ensure proper muscular development and to reduce your risk of injury. Only in sport-specific training programs should you consider changing the speed of an exercise movement.

The musculoskeletal system moves through a specific range of motion when the brain sends nerve impulses that stimulate muscles to move bones and body parts.

The following sections describe the ranges of motion, including extension, flexion, hyperextension, hyperflexion, and more. Table 4.3 lists all the various joint movements.

Table 4.3 **Joint Movements of the Human Body**

Joint Movement	Description
Extension	Occurs when a joint's range of motion is moving towards an end point of 0 degrees (refer to "Extension" following this table).
Flexion	Occurs when a joint's range of motion is moving towards an end point of 180 degrees (refer to "Flexion" later in this chapter).
Hyperextension	The joint is forced past a 0-degree range of motion, usually resulting in injury to the joint's tendons and/or ligaments.
Hyperflexion	The excessive bending of a joint beyond its normal anatomical position, usually resulting in injury to the joint's tendons and/or ligaments.
Dorsiflexion	Occurs when the ankle joint's range of motion is moving towards an end point of 90 degrees. In simple terms, dorsiflexion means "bending the foot upward."
Plantar flexion	Occurs when the ankle joint's range of motion is moving towards an end point of 45 degrees. In simple terms, plantar flexion means "pointing the toes downward."
Circumduction	The circular rotation motion of a joint.
Supination	Turning the palm upwards.
Pronation	Turning the palm downward.
Inversion	Turning the foot so the sole is inward.
Eversion	Turning the foot so the sole is outward.
Abduction	Moving the body parts and joints away from the midline of the body.
Shoulder abduction (acromionclavicular joint)	The acromionclavicular joint is abducting when the medial deltoid muscle performs the upward (lifting outward) movement during the side lateral raise exercise.
Hip abduction	The hip socket is abducting when the tensor fascia latae muscle performs the outward movement from a standing position during the hip abduction exercise.
Adduction	Moving the body parts and joints towards the midline of the body.
Shoulder adduction (acromionclavicular joint)	The acromionclavicular joint is adducting when the medial deltoid muscle performs the downward (lifting outward) movement during the side lateral raise exercise.

Table 4.3   **Joint Movements of the Human Body (Continued)**

Hip adduction	The hip socket is abducting when the tensor fascia latae muscle performs the inward movement from a standing position during the hip abduction exercise.
Protraction	Moving a body part into forward motion. An example of protraction is moving the head forward.
Retraction	Moving a body part in a backward direction. An example of retraction is pulling the head backwards.
Rotation	Moving a body part in a pivotal axis motion. An example of rotation is moving your head from the left to the right.
Elevation	Raising a body part upward. An example of elevation is shrugging the trapezius muscles.
Depression	Lowering a body part. An example of depression is relaxing the trapezius muscles.

Extension

Extension occurs when a joint's range of motion is moving towards an end point of 0 degrees. In other words, extension means straightening the joint and increasing the angle between the body parts that are moving. Extension occurs within certain joints of the body, as described here:

■ Knee extension (patella femoral joint)—The patella femoral joint is extending when the quadriceps muscles perform the upward movement during the quadriceps leg extension exercise.

■ Elbow extension (radioulnar joint)—The radioulnar joint is extending when the triceps muscles perform the downward (pressing) movement during the triceps pushdown exercise.

■ Wrist joint extension (radiocarpal)—The radiocarpal joint is extending when the top of the hand is moving towards the body during a wrist curl exercise.

■ Shoulder extension (acromionclavicular joint)—The acromionclavicular joint is extending when the deltoid muscle performs the overhead pressing movement during the seated shoulder press exercise.

■ Lumbar spine extension (sacroiliac joint)—The sacroiliac joint is extending when the erector spinae muscles perform the upward movement during a lower back extension exercise.

■ Hip extension (hip socket)—The hip socket is extending when the quadratus lumborum muscle and gluteal muscles perform a backwards movement (foot behind the body) from a standing position during the hip extension exercise.

Flexion

Flexion occurs when a joint's range of motion is moving towards an end point of 180 degrees. In other words, flexion means bending the joint and decreasing the angle between the body parts that are moving. Flexion occurs within certain joints of the body, as described below:

- Knee flexion (patella femoral joint)—The patella femoral joint is flexing when the hamstrings muscles perform the upward movement during the hamstrings leg curl exercise.

- Elbow flexion (radioulnar joint)—The radioulnar joint is flexing when the biceps brachii muscles perform the upward movement during the dumbell biceps curl exercise.

- Wrist joint flexion (radiocarpal)—The radiocarpal joint is flexing when the palm is moving towards the body during a wrist curl exercise.

- Shoulder flexion (acromionclavicular joint)—The acromionclavicular joint is flexing when the deltoid muscles perform the downward movement during the seated shoulder press exercise.

- Lumbar spine flexion (sacroiliac joint)—The sacroiliac joint is flexing when the erector spinae muscles perform the downward movement during the lower back extension exercise.

- Hip flexion (hip socket)—The hip socket is flexing when the illio psoas muscle and sartorius muscle perform the forward movement (foot in front of the body) from a standing position during the hip flexion exercise.

Exercise Movements

Three terms describe a muscle's movement during a resistive strength training exercise: isotonic movement, isokinetic movement, and isometric movement.

An isotonic exercise movement involves moving a constant weight volume during a controlled range of motion at a controlled speed, which is relatively slow. The resistance of weight volume does not change during the entire strength curve (the muscle's strength range from the beginning to the end of the exercise movement).

An example of an isotonic exercise is performing a barbell chest press for ten repetitions with 135 pounds of weight. Throughout the ten repetitions, the full range of motion is performed, the resistance stays constant, and the strength curve of the exercise movement does not change.

An isokinetic exercise movement involves moving a varied weight volume during a controlled range of motion at different fixed speeds (slow or fast). The resistance of weight volume changes during the entire strength curve. Isokinetic exercises are referred to as "accommodating resistance" exercises.

An example of an isokinetic exercise is performing a side lateral raise using a therapy band for ten repetitions. Throughout the ten repetitions, the full range of motion stays constant and the speed is constant, but the resistance changes due to the elasticity of the therapy band. The therapy band creates a greater amount of resistance during the concentric contraction because it is stretched further. The therapy band creates less resistance during the eccentric contraction because it is not stretched to its fullest length. The greater the force applied to the therapy band, the greater the resistance.

An isometric exercise movement involves a weight volume that stays constant during the exercise. The entire strength curve is static.

An example of an isometric exercise movement is a body weight wall sit (sitting in a static position against a wall without a chair's support for a period of time). Throughout the entire exercise, the volume of resistance (body weight) stays constant, and there is no movement.

Muscles that are used in an exercise movement are referred to as the agonist, antagonist, and synergist muscles.

- The agonist is the muscle being used in an exercise movement. The agonist is the primary mover. For example, the biceps femoris muscle is the agonist during the hamstrings leg curl exercise.

- The antagonist is the opposing muscle of the primary mover that is being used in the exercise movement. For example, the rectus femoris muscle is the antagonist during the hamstrings leg curl exercise.

- The synergist, or secondary muscle, is the stabilizing or assisting muscle group or groups being used along with the agonist and antagonist muscles during the exercise movement. For example, the triceps muscle group is the synergist assisting the deltoid muscles during the seated shoulder press exercise.

Muscle Physiology

Understanding something about muscle physiology should help you understand kinesiology.

Muscular endurance is your muscle's ability to withstand isolated or overall effects of fatigue during a movement. To increase your muscular endurance, you need to use light to moderate volumes of weight with maximal repetitions during a specific exercise. For instance, you could increase your number of repetitions while lifting 120 pounds during a barbell chest press.

Muscular strength is the measurement of increases in absolute muscular power (overall strength) and speed in the muscle during a movement. To increase your muscular strength, you need to use increasingly heavy volumes of weight with minimal repetitions during a specific exercise. For example, you could lift 120 pounds for ten repetitions during the first set of the barbell chest press exercise, and then increase that to 180 pounds for ten repetitions during your second set.

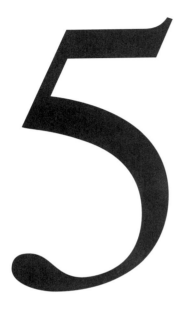

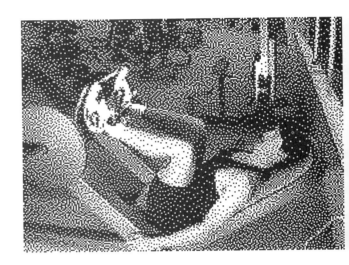

Planning Your
Fitness Program

THIS CHAPTER GIVES YOU AN OVERVIEW OF HOW TO DESIGN YOUR FITNESS program. It explains what types of stretching, strength training, and cardiovascular routines will fit your needs, depending upon both your current level of fitness and your fitness goals. It also supplies you with sound advice for warding off injuries, as well as for handling injuries when they do occur. Finally, it provides you with some quick tips about measuring your progress, a good way to both motivate yourself and to check whether your fitness program is doing its intended job.

Preventing and Treating Injuries

Whenever you exercise, you should take some simple precautions to reduce the risk of injuring yourself. If misfortunately you suffer an injury, you should immediately consult a physician or your health care provider. At the same time, there are a few easy steps you can follow to take good care of your injury, as you'll learn shortly.

Preventing Injuries

When participating in a fitness program, warming up and cooling down are the surest ways to avoid injuring yourself. The best way to prevent injuries is to ensure that your strength and cardiovascular exercises involve these four phases:

- Warm-up phase

- Training phase

- Cool-down phase

- Flexibility phase

Warm-up Phase

Any time you engage in physical activity, you should begin with the proper warm-up, which will elevate your core temperature, elevate your heart rate, and bring oxygen and blood flow to the specific muscles you'll be using in the exercise. As you warm up, make sure to move the larger muscle groups in a slow, controlled range of motion at a low heart rate intensity for 5 to 10 minutes. For example, you could warm up by performing light cycling, walking, light jogging, arm circles, or gentle stretching.

Training Phase

The training phase follows the warm-up phase. During this phase, you actually perform the cardiovascular exercise and/or strength training activity.

Cool-down Phase

After the training phase comes the cool-down phase, during which you decrease your body core temperature and level of heart rate intensity to properly prepare your body for the end of your training program. The American College of Sports Medicine recommends that you decrease your heart rate level to 100 beats per minute or less to conclude your exercise workout. Perform the cool-down phase for 2 to 5 minutes after the training phase.

The cool-down phase helps to prevent blood pooling and lactic acid deposits in your muscle groups. Cooling down properly will decrease your level of muscular soreness as well as any possible coronary artery risks that may be associated with cardiovascular exercise.

Flexibility Phase

After the cool-down phase comes the flexibility phase (stretching). You should stretch the muscle groups that you used during an exercise to

- Increase the range of motion within the joints and muscles.

- Elongate muscle groups and allow the muscles to grow more efficiently.

- Decrease your risk of injury.

See the section "Stretching and Flexibility" later in this chapter.

Treating Injuries

If you follow the preceding precautions, you're less likely to injure yourself while exercising. But injuries do happen. This section explains what to do if you're injured, and describes how to care for your injuries to aid the healing process.

If you injure yourself, consult a physician or health care professional immediately to get an accurate diagnosis for care. In addition, most athletic and nonathletic related injuries can benefit from the four easy steps described next. These steps are sometimes abbreviated as the acronym RICE, which represents the following:

- **Rest (R)**   Rest the injured body part for a certain period of time depending upon the condition of the injury. You may have to take a day off from work, use crutches, or simply refrain from participating in the activity that caused the injury.

- **Ice (I)**   Ice (cold compress) is the best remedy for most injuries. 95 percent of injury cases require immediate application of a cold compress—ice inside a plastic bag wrapped in a towel or paper towel.

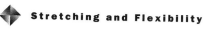

Directly apply the cold compress to the injured area to decrease the amount of swelling or internal bleeding following a contusion or other musculoskeletal injury. The cold compress can significantly decrease the amount of pain, swelling, and muscle spasm in the injured area. A cold compress can also help you more quickly recover from your injury and return to normal activity.

When applying ice, you can use simple ice bags, commercial ice packs, or ice massage; or in some cases, you can completely immerse the injured area in ice. You can apply a cold compress for periods of up to 20 minutes (but no more), and you should not use a cold compress for more than two such intervals in an hour.

You can use a cold compress for up to 72 hours immediately following an injury, and can use it thereafter with localized swelling. If the pain and swelling do not decrease after 72 hours, please consult your physician or health care provider.

- **Compression (C)** Compression involves applying an elastic bandage to the injured area to control swelling or edema. When applying a compression bandage, make sure that the wrap is not too tight, or you may impair circulation.

- **Elevation (E)** Elevation simply means using gravity to minimize swelling and to support venous and lymphatic circulation. This process facilitates removal of waste products associated with trauma and encourages the return to normal circulation.

Stretching and Flexibility

Stretching exercises enable you to develop greater ranges of motion in your muscles and joints, helping you avoid injury. Taking the time to increase your flexibility also elongates your muscle groups, which, in turn, helps to produce greater muscle size and muscle strength. For these reasons, you should incorporate a consistent regimen of stretching and flexibility exercises into any strength training routine and/or cardiovascular training routine.

Before stretching, remember to warm up for 5 to 10 minutes to increase your body's core temperature and increase blood flow to your muscles. Bicycling, walking, skipping rope, and other moderate activities are good warm-up exercises. Also remember to stretch after concluding your exercise session. This helps you to achieve greater muscle growth and reduces muscle soreness and risk of injury.

There are two basic types of stretches: static stretches and ballistic stretches. During a *static stretch*, you apply constant resistance against the affected muscle groups and skeletal joints in a safe and controlled range of motion. You should perform static stretches for 10 to 30 seconds per stretch. If you like, you can stretch a certain muscle group area more than once.

During a *ballistic stretch*, you perform a "bouncing" type of movement while stretching the affected muscle groups and skeletal joints in a short range of motion at a moderate to fast pace. Any stretch movement that incorporates "bouncing" tends to shorten and lengthen the affected muscles for too short a time period, creating a "rubber band" effect upon the skeletal joints and muscle groups. Ballistic stretches are not considered biomechanically correct; they actually increase your risk of injury and do not enhance the flexibility of your skeletal joints and muscle groups. For this reason, such stretches are not recommended.

Strength Training

Strength training is a critical component of any fitness program. Properly implemented, a strength training program increases your muscular strength, muscular endurance, muscle mass (lean body mass), muscle definition, muscle cell size (hypertrophy), bone density, and the efficiency of your metabolism. It also reduces your risk of musculoskeletal injury and develops your overall physique.

You need to weigh a number of factors when designing a suitable strength training routine. First, you must consider your current level of fitness. Second, you need to determine which muscle groups you want to exercise. And finally, you have to calculate precisely how to exercise each selected muscle group, deciding which exercises to perform, how many repetitions to carry out, how much weight to lift, and more.

Make sure to consider your health history and any physical limitations or injuries when designing a strength training program. You can use the baseline statistics and information from your personal fitness assessment (see Chapter 3 or the "Getting Started" section on the CD-ROM) to determine your health and fitness levels. The three fitness levels are

- Beginning fitness level (B)

- Intermediate fitness level (I)

- Advanced fitness level (A)

Designing a safe and effective strength training program also involves selecting which muscles to strengthen and in what order to strengthen them. The best way to strength train is to strengthen the larger muscle groups first, and then strengthen the smaller muscle groups. For example, if you were working out your lower body, you would exercise your gluteals before your quadriceps, and your quadriceps before your calves. The following lists divide the body into three planes—lower body, upper body, and abdominals and lower back. Within each category, the muscle groups are listed in order from largest to smallest.

I. Lower Body

1. Gluteal muscles group (buttocks)

2. Hip muscles group (psoas, adductors, and abductors)

3. Quadriceps muscles group (vastus medialis, vastus lateralis, vastus intermedius, and rectus femoris)

4. Hamstrings muscles group (semimembranosis, semitendinosis, and biceps femoris)

5. Calf muscle group (soleus, gastrocnemius, anterior tibialis)

II. Upper Body

1. Chest (pectoralis major and pectoralis minor)

2. Upper back (latissimus dorsi and rhomboids)

3. Shoulders (anterior, medial and posterior deltoid, and trapezius)

4. Rotator cuff (supraspinatus, infraspinatus, teres major and minor, and subscapularis)

5. Triceps (long, medium, and short heads)

6. Biceps (biceps brachii, brachiallis, and brachioradialis)

7. Forearms (flexors and extensors)

III. Abdominals and Lower Back

1. Abdominals (transverse and rectus abdominus, and obliques)

2. Lower back (quadratus lumborum and erector spinae)

You should exercise your abdominal and lower-back muscle groups at the end of your exercise routine. If you exercise these muscle groups first, you'll "prefatigue" the mid-torso area, possibly increasing your risk for injury.

Finally, when implementing a strength training routine, you need to take into consideration the following factors:

- Exercise selection

- Set selection

- Repetition selection

- Intensity
- Duration
- Training frequency
- Rest

Each of these components is discussed in more detail in the sections that follow.

Exercise Selection

Exercise selection simply means choosing how many and which exercises to carry out for each muscle group. It's also important to carry out your exercises in the proper sequence.

Number of Exercises per Muscle Group

The number of exercises you perform for each body part naturally depends upon your fitness level.

- Beginners should choose one exercise per muscle group.
- Intermediate exercisers should choose two to three exercises per muscle group.
- Advanced exercisers should choose three to five exercises per muscle group.

You should also choose exercises based upon the results you want from your strength training program.

- One exercise per muscle group enhances muscular adaptation.
- Two to three exercises per muscle group enhances muscular strength and muscular endurance.
- Three to five exercises per muscle group enhances muscular strength and muscular power.

You should perform anywhere from one to five exercises for the larger muscle groups, including the legs (quadriceps and hamstrings), the hips and buttocks (iliopsoas, adductors, abductors and gluteals), the chest (pectoralis major and pectoralis minor), the upper back (latissimus dorsi and rhomboids), and the shoulders (anterior, medial and posterior deltoid, and trapezius)

You should perform anywhere from one to four exercises for the smaller muscle groups, including the rotator cuff (supraspinatus, infraspinatus, teres major, and subscapularis), the triceps (long, medium, and short heads), the biceps (biceps brachii, brachialis, and brachioradialis), the forearms (flexors and extensors), and the calves (soleus, gastrocnemius, and anterior tibialis).

You should perform anywhere from one to five exercises for the abdominal muscles (transverse and rectus abdominus, and obliques) and the lower back muscle groups (quadratus lumborum and erector spinae).

Types of Exercises

The type of exercise you select for your strength training program depends upon your fitness level and strength goals. There are two basic categories of strength training exercises, individual muscle exercises and multiple muscle exercises.

Individual Muscle Exercise (Single Joint Movement)

An exercise that emphasizes only one muscle group (called the primary muscle) and moves only one skeletal joint is called an individual muscle exercise or a single joint movement exercise.

An example of an individual muscle exercise is a dumbbell biceps curl. The biceps muscle is emphasized as the primary muscle. The single joint that moves is the elbow joint, which is flexing and extending throughout the exercise.

Multiple Muscle Exercise (Multiple Joint Movement)

An exercise that emphasizes multiple muscle groups (called the primary muscle and the secondary muscles) and moves more than one skeletal joint is called a multiple muscle exercise or multiple joint movement exercise.

For example, a barbell chest press is a multiple muscle exercise. It emphasizes the chest muscles (the primary muscle), as well as the shoulder muscles and triceps muscles (the secondary muscles). The two joints that are moving during the exercise are the elbow joint and the shoulder joint. The elbow joint is flexing and extending and the shoulder joint is abducting and adducting.

Performing Exercises in the Proper Sequence

It's vital to perform your exercises in the proper sequence while strength training. If you're a beginning or intermediate level exerciser, you should carry out multiple muscle exercises before performing individual muscle exercises. It's more challenging to do the reverse: performing individual muscle exercises before engaging in multiple muscle exercises. This sequence is recommended for advanced strength training routines only.

Performing individual muscle exercises before multiple muscle exercises prefatigues the individual muscle that might stabilize the secondary muscle group being strengthened during the next exercise. For beginners, prefatiguing a muscle could lead to possible injury and may also create a negative result in overall strength gains. If you're at an advanced fitness level, you can consider preexhausting muscles; otherwise, you should confine yourself to performing multiple muscle exercises before individual muscle exercises.

Set Selection

As you can probably guess, set selection refers to the number of times that you perform the exercise. For example, you might determine that you need to perform three sets of ten repetitions apiece. (Repetition selection is covered a bit later in the chapter.) In addition, there are different types of sets, as you'll learn in a moment. The number of sets you perform for each exercise depends upon your fitness level.

- Beginners should perform one set per exercise.

- Intermediate exercisers should perform two to three sets per exercise.

- Advanced exercisers should perform three to five sets per exercise.

You should also base the number of sets you perform upon the desired results of your strength training program.

- Perform one set per exercise for muscular adaptation.

- Perform two to three sets per exercise selection for muscular strength and muscular endurance gains.

- Perform three to five sets per exercise selection for muscular strength and power gains.

There are many types of strength training sets that you can incorporate into a strength training sequence, including standard sets, staggered sets, pyramid sets, strip sets, and priority principle sets.

Standard Set

A standard set is a sequence in which you perform the same strength training exercise with a rest period of 30 to 90 seconds between sets. You can include standard sets in any strength training exercise sequence; such sets are recommended for exercisers at all fitness levels.

Here is a standard set in which you use the chest, shoulders, and triceps muscles by performing a dumbbell flat chest press.

Exercise	Repetitions	Sets	Weight Volume
Dumbbell Flat Chest Press	6–10	2–3	Moderate-Heavy
Rest			
Dumbbell Flat Chest Press	6–10	2–3	Moderate-Heavy
Rest			
Dumbbell Flat Chest Press	6–10	2–3	Moderate-Heavy

Staggered Set

In a staggered set, you perform a strength training exercise for the biceps or triceps muscle in between performing a larger muscle group exercise. You should perform an individual muscle exercise for the biceps muscle or triceps muscle in between performing a multiple muscle exercise for the larger muscle group.

A staggered set is a great way to preexhaust and post exhaust the stabilizing muscle groups of the body. You can incorporate a staggered set in any strength training exercise sequence, but these types of sets are recommended only for exercisers at an advanced level of fitness.

Here is a staggered set that implements a triceps exercise in between a chest exercise. Perform a dumbbell triceps extension exercise in between the barbell flat chest press exercise.

Exercise	Repetitions	Sets	Weight Volume
Dumbbell Triceps Extension	6–10	1	Moderate-Heavy
Barbell Flat Chest Press	6–10	1	Moderate-Heavy
Dumbbell Triceps Extension	6–10	1	Moderate-Heavy
Barbell Flat Chest Press	6–10	1	Moderate-Heavy
Dumbbell Triceps Extension	6–10	1	Moderate-Heavy
Barbell Flat Chest Press	6–10	1	Moderate-Heavy

Pyramid Set

In a pyramid set, you increase or decrease the number of repetitions you perform in each exercise set while increasing or decreasing the weight volume. Increasing the repetitions and decreasing the weight volume enhances muscular endurance. Decreasing the repetitions while increasing the weight volume enhances muscular strength. You can incorporate a pyramid set into any strength training exercise sequence, but these types of sets are recommended only for exercisers at an advanced fitness level.

There are actually two types of pyramid sets: the muscular strength pyramid set and the muscular endurance pyramid set. In a muscular strength pyramid set, you decrease the number of repetitions that you perform in each exercise set while simultaneously increasing the volume of weight. A muscular strength pyramid set is composed of four sets for one strength training exercise. Each set increases approximately 10 percent in weight volume intensity and decreases the number of repetitions by two.

Here is a muscular strength pyramid set for the chest muscles. You perform the barbell flat chest press for four sets.

Exercise	Repetitions	Sets	Weight Volume
Barbell Flat Chest Press	10	1	135 lbs.
Barbell Flat Chest Press	8	1	150 lbs.
Barbell Flat Chest Press	6	1	165 lbs.
Barbell Flat Chest Press	4	1	180 lbs.

In a muscular endurance pyramid set, in contrast, you increase the number of repetitions that you perform in each exercise set while decreasing the volume of weight. A muscular endurance pyramid set is composed of four sets for one strength training exercise. Each set decreases approximately 10 percent in weight volume intensity and increases the number of repetitions by two.

Here is a muscular endurance pyramid set for the chest muscles. Perform the barbell flat chest press for four sets.

Exercise	Repetitions	Sets	Weight Volume
Barbell Flat Chest Press	8	1	180 lbs.
Barbell Flat Chest Press	10	1	165 lbs.
Barbell Flat Chest Press	12	1	150 lbs.
Barbell Flat Chest Press	14	1	135 lbs.

Strip Set

In a strip set, you perform a strength training exercise with the greatest possible weight volume for eight to ten repetitions or until you achieve muscular failure (exhaustion). At this point, you decrease the weight volume by 5 to 10 percent and perform the next set of the same strength training exercise immediately for another eight to ten repetitions or until you achieve muscular failure.

You repeat the strip set routine until you can no longer perform any repetitions of the strength training exercise or you reach the lightest weight volume. There is no rest between the strip sets. The point of strip sets is to increase muscular endurance and overload the muscles being strengthened. You can include strip sets in any strength training exercise sequence, but they are recommended only for exercisers who are at an advanced level of fitness.

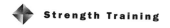

There are three types of strip set routines:

■ The weight machine strip set

■ The barbell strip set

■ The dumbbell strip set

When using the weight machine, begin the strip set routine with the heaviest weight that you can lift for eight to ten repetitions. After you achieve muscular failure with the beginning weight volume, lighten the weight (move the pin up the stack) and perform as many repetitions as possible until you reach muscular failure at the new weight volume. Continue in this manner—performing repetitions until you reach muscular failure—at each weight volume until you reach the lightest setting of weight volume on the weight stack.

Here is an example strip set for the chest muscles. You perform the machine chest press for ten sets. If you can begin at a higher weight volume, you of course will have to perform additional sets.

Exercise	Repetitions	Sets	Weight Volume
Machine Chest Press	8–10	1	100 lbs.
Machine Chest Press	8–10	1	90 lbs.
Machine Chest Press	8–10	1	80 lbs.
Machine Chest Press	8–10	1	70 lbs.
Machine Chest Press	8–10	1	60 lbs.
Machine Chest Press	8–10	1	50 lbs.
Machine Chest Press	8–10	1	40 lbs.
Machine Chest Press	8–10	1	30 lbs.
Machine Chest Press	8–10	1	20 lbs.
Machine Chest Press	8–10	1	10 lbs.

When using barbells, begin the strip set routine with the heaviest weight that you can lift for eight to ten repetitions. After you achieve muscular failure with the beginning weight volume, remove the weight plates from the barbell in increments of 10 to 20 percent per strip set (lightening the weight) and perform as many repetitions as possible until you reach muscular failure at the new weight volume. Continue in this manner—performing repetitions until you reach muscular failure—at each weight volume until there is no additional weight left on the barbell.

Here is an example strip set for the chest muscles. You perform the barbell incline chest press for nine sets. If you can begin at a higher weight volume, you must perform additional sets to complete the exercise.

Exercise	Repetitions	Sets	Weight Volume
Barbell Incline Chest Press	8–10	1	130 lbs.
Barbell Incline Chest Press	8–10	1	115 lbs.
Barbell Incline Chest Press	8–10	1	105 lbs.
Barbell Incline Chest Press	8–10	1	95 lbs.
Barbell Incline Chest Press	8–10	1	85 lbs.
Barbell Incline Chest Press	8–10	1	75 lbs.
Barbell Incline Chest Press	8–10	1	65 lbs.
Barbell Incline Chest Press	8–10	1	55 lbs.
Barbell Incline Chest Press	8–10	1	45 lbs.

When using dumbbells, begin the strip set routine with the heaviest dumbbell that you can lift for eight to ten repetitions. After muscular failure occurs with the beginning weight volume, decrease the weight volume of the dumbbell by 5 percent (lightening the weight) and perform as many repetitions as possible until you achieve muscular failure at the new weight volume. Continue in this manner—performing repetitions until you reach muscular failure—at each weight volume until you use the lightest dumbbell on the rack. This is termed "running the rack."

Here is an example strip set for the shoulder muscles. In this case, you perform the dumbbell shoulder press for nine sets. If you can begin at a higher weight volume, you need to perform additional sets to complete the exercise.

Exercise	Repetitions	Sets	Weight Volume
Dumbbell Shoulder Press	8–10	1	45 lbs.
Dumbbell Shoulder Press	8–10	1	40 lbs.

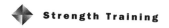

Dumbbell Shoulder Press	8–10	1	35 lbs.
Dumbbell Shoulder Press	8–10	1	30 lbs.
Dumbbell Shoulder Press	8–10	1	25 lbs.
Dumbbell Shoulder Press	8–10	1	20 lbs.
Dumbbell Shoulder Press	8–10	1	15 lbs.
Dumbbell Shoulder Press	8–10	1	10 lbs.
Dumbbell Shoulder Press	8–10	1	5 lbs.

Priority Principle Set

The priority principle set focuses on training the weaker muscle groups at the beginning of the strength training routine, when the body is strongest. You shouldn't perform a priority principle set during a full body workout, when it may increase your risk of injury.

A priority principle set is recommended only for advanced fitness level exercisers and should be implemented into split routines for different muscle groups only.

Here's an example of a priority principle set that strengthens the biceps before using them in a multijoint back exercise movement.

Exercise	Repetitions	Sets	Weight Volume
Barbell Biceps Curl	8–12	2–3	Moderate-Heavy
Dumbbell Biceps Curl	8–12	2–3	Moderate-Heavy
Barbell Reverse Curl	8–12	2–3	Moderate-Heavy
Rear Pulldown	8-12	2-3	Moderate-Heavy
Front Pulldown	8-12	2-3	Moderate-Heavy
Dumbbell Row	8-12	2-3	Moderate-Heavy

Repetition Selection

Repetition selection refers to the number of times that you perform the exercise movement during the set. The number of repetitions you perform affects your muscular strength, muscular endurance, and muscular hypertrophy (size).

If you are beginning a strength training program, you should start out with 15 to 20 repetitions for the first three weeks of your program. After completing the first three weeks, you should choose one of the following repetition ranges, depending upon your fitness level and desired strength goals.

- Beginners should perform 12 to 20 repetitions.

- Intermediate exercisers should perform 8 to 12 repetitions.

- Advanced exercisers should perform 6 to 8 repetitions.

You should also base your repetition selection upon the results you want from your strength training program.

- Performing 12 to 20 repetitions will produce muscular endurance gains and muscle hypertrophy (increase in muscle cell size).

- Performing 8 to 12 repetitions will yield muscular strength and muscular endurance gains.

- Performing 6 to 8 repetitions will result in muscular strength and power gains.

Intensity

Intensity refers to the amount of weight volume (pounds) that you use during a strength training exercise activity. You should select a weight volume based upon your fitness level and your goals for strength improvement. The amount of weight you lift affects your muscular strength, muscular endurance, and muscular hypertrophy (size).

To determine the correct amount of weight volume to use for an exercise set, you must first determine your one repetition maximum for that exercise movement. A one repetition maximum refers to the greatest amount of weight that you can lift one time.

Lifting the maximum weight that you can one time can be dangerous to your joints, ligaments, and tendons, especially if you are a beginner. A safe way to *estimate* a one repetition maximum is to perform an exercise for 10 repetitions with an amount of weight that you believe will exhaust your muscles within 10 repetitions. If you do not have any idea what this weight amount should be, then you should use a weight volume that is equal to 25 percent (men) or 15 percent (women) of your body weight to begin with and build up from there.

If you can perform this exercise (with proper form and motion) for more than 10 repetitions with the weight used, rest for 2–3 minutes and increase the weight load you just used by 5–10 percent for the next set of repetitions. Continue to increase the weight load until you find a weight that exhausts your muscles within 10 repetitions.

After the 10 repetitions are performed and the muscle is exhausted, use this formula to determine your estimated one repetition maximum:

Pounds of weight lifted 10 times divided by 0.75 = one repetition maximum

For example, a barbell flat chest press is performed with 150 pounds for 10 repetitions. Your estimated one repetition maximum is 200 pounds (150 ÷ 0.75). Determining a one repetition maximum for each exercise is a safe way to determine the correct weight volume for each upper- and lower-body exercise in your strength training routine.

Fitness Level and Strength Goals

Weight volume selection is based upon your level of fitness and your strength goals.

■ A light level of weight volume is 40–60 percent of your one repetition maximum. This weight volume selection is recommended for beginner fitness level exercisers and is generally used to increase muscular endurance. Increasing the weight volume 0–5 percent for each set is recommended when using a light weight volume during an exercise.

■ A moderate level of weight volume is 60–80 percent of your one repetition maximum. This weight volume is recommended for intermediate and advanced fitness level exercisers and is generally used to produce muscular strength and muscular endurance. Increasing the weight volume 5–10 percent for each set is recommended when using a moderate weight volume during an exercise.

■ A heavy level of weight volume is 80–100 percent of your one repetition maximum. This weight volume is recommended for advanced fitness level exercisers and is used generally to increase muscular power and strength. Increasing the weight volume 10–15 percent for each set is recommended when using a heavy weight volume during an exercise.

You should also base the amount of weight you lift on the results you want from your strength training program.

■ For muscular endurance gains, use a light intensity of weight volume increase (0 to 5 percent per set).

■ For muscular strength and muscular endurance gains, use a moderate intensity of weight volume increase (5 to 10 percent per set).

■ For muscular strength and power gains, use a heavy intensity of weight volume increase (10 to 15 percent per set).

Duration

Duration refers to the period of time, in minutes, that you exercise with weights during your strength training program. (Duration is not the same as training frequency, which refers to the number of days per week that you exercise, as described in a moment.)

The American College of Sports Medicine recommends a minimum of 20 minutes of strength training to achieve any increases in muscular strength, muscular endurance, muscle mass, and bone density, as well as changes in your metabolic system. The length of time that you exercise will depend upon your fitness level.

- Beginners should perform strength training exercises for 20 minutes.

- Intermediate exercisers should perform strength training exercises for 20 to 40 minutes.

- Advanced exercisers should perform strength training exercises for 40 to 60 minutes.

If you are training for a specific sporting event or are an elite-level athlete (college and professional), you should strength train for over 60 minutes. The exact amount of time will depend upon your health and fitness goals.

Training Frequency

Training frequency refers to the number of days per week that you strength train. The American College of Sports Medicine recommends strength training for a minimum of two to three days per week to achieve any increases in muscular strength, muscular endurance, muscle mass, and bone density, as well as changes in your metabolic system. The number of days per week you should strength train depends upon your fitness level.

- Beginners should train two to three days per week.

- Intermediate exercisers should train three to four days per week.

- Advanced exercisers should train five to six days per week.

Rest

Any fitness program should include at least one total rest day (no activity). Resting the musculoskeletal system allows the body to recover and regenerate its energy level. Strength training consistently without any rest can lead to musculoskeletal injury.

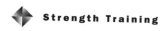
At What Level Should You Strength Train?

When should you increase the difficulty level of your strength training program? The simple answer is when it becomes too easy. You should move on to a more challenging routine if, when performing your routine, you can comfortably perform

- The selected exercises

- The selected sets

- The selected repetitions

- The selected intensity

- The selected duration

- The selected training frequency

You should change your strength training routine—the exercises, the number of sets, the number of repetitions, the intensity, and so forth—every three to four weeks to enhance muscular strength, muscular endurance, and muscle size.

If your strength training program is too easy you won't make progress. But your program should not be too difficult either, or you risk overtraining. Overtraining with weights means strength training without following the proper guidelines for your individual fitness level and health goals. Overtraining can be detrimental to your musculoskeletal system, overall strength, and exercise participation. It can also increase your risk for musculoskeletal injury and can adversely affect your mental and physical state. These are some of the signs of overtraining:

- Injury

- Trouble sleeping

- Decreased desire to participate

- Decreased appetite

- Irritability

- Unable to increase fitness goals

If you experience any of these symptoms, please reevaluate your strength training program, making sure that you're not lifting too much weight too often, resting insufficiently, and the like. Keep in mind that any strength training activity should include an appropriate warm-up period, cool-down period, and subsequent flexibility exercises. See the section "Preventing and Treating Injuries" earlier in this chapter for the details.

Cardiovascular Training

A properly designed cardiovascular training program should increase your level of maximal oxygen uptake (aerobic or V02 capacity). To devise a safe and effective cardiovascular training program, you need to consider the results of your V02 test in the personal fitness assessment (see Chapter 3) as well as your specific fitness goals.

The general health and fitness goals of a cardiovascular program are

- Cardiovascular improvement

- Weight loss and body fat reduction

- Increased muscular endurance

- Reduction of coronary artery disease

Like a strength training routine, a cardiovascular exercise routine should include an appropriate warm-up period, cool-down period, and subsequent flexibility exercises. See the section "Preventing and Treating Injuries" earlier in this chapter for the details.

Determining the Correct Target Heart Rate Range

To design an effective cardiovascular program, you must determine your correct estimated target heart rate level and V02 capacity level. Consult Chapter 3 for the details on how to calculate both your age-predicted maximal heart rate and your karvonen training heart rate level.

Your age-predicted maximal heart rate level is the level at which your heart is estimated to be working (measured in beats per minute) at the highest level (100 percent) while you are performing a cardiovascular exercise. The estimated maximal heart rate level (100 percent) is determined by your age. The American College of Sports Medicine recommends that you maintain a target heart rate range of 50 to 90 percent of your age-predicted maximal heart rate when performing an aerobic exercise.

- The 50- to 60-percent age-predicted maximal heart rate range increases the body's metabolic rate, but is unlikely to result in cardiovascular improvement. This heart rate range is recommended for beginning exercisers.

- The 60- to 85-percent age-predicted maximal heart rate range will help you achieve cardiovascular improvement and body fat loss. This heart rate range is recommended for intermediate to advanced level exercisers.

- The 85- to 90-percent age-predicted maximal heart rate range is recommended for advanced fitness level exercisers only.

■ Only elite fitness level athletes should perform an aerobic exercise above their 90-percent age-predicted maximal heart rate level.

Your Karvonen training heart rate level is the level at which your heart rate is estimated to be working at the most effective aerobic training heart rate range while performing a cardiovascular exercise. The Karvonen training heart rate level is determined by your age and resting heart rate measurement. Exercising within 60 to 80 percent of the target heart rate range of age-predicted heart rate is the safest and most effective way to improve the cardiovascular system and increase your aerobic capacity. For determining your age-predicted heart rate or Karvonen heart rate, refer to Chapter 3.

Rate of Perceived Exertion (RPE) Scale

The rate of perceived exertion (RPE) scale helps you measure your estimated level of aerobic exercise by how you feel during your cardiovascular exercise routine. This scale (shown in Table 5.1) gives you a point of reference for determining whether you are exercising too hard or not hard enough. Most people should exercise between 3 (moderate) and 7 (very hard) on the scale throughout their routine.

The FIT Principle for Cardiovascular Exercise

FIT is short for "frequency," "intensity," and "time." These components should figure into the design of any cardiovascular exercise program.

Frequency

Frequency is simply the number of times per week that you perform a cardiovascular exercise activity. The American College of Sports Medicine recommends performing an aerobic exercise three times per week to improve your cardiovascular system's aerobic capacity, stimulate body fat reduction and weight loss, and increase your basal metabolic rate. Increasing the frequency with which you exercise to five to six times per week will produce even greater improvements to your cardiovascular system and musculoskeletal system.

Always include a total rest day (no activity) in your cardiovascular exercise program.

Intensity

Intensity refers to your heart rate level, V02 (oxygen uptake) capacity level, and rate of perceived exertion (RPE) scale level during a cardiovascular exercise activity. Refer to the sections "Determining the Correct Target Heart Rate Range" and "Rate of Perceived Exertion (RPE) Scale" in this chapter, as well as Chapter 3 for additional details on monitoring your heart rate level as well as your rate of perceived exertion.

Table 5.1	**RPE Scale**

RPE Level	Difficulty
10	Maximal, can do no more
09	
08	Very hard
07	
06	Harder
05	Hard
04	More difficult
03	Moderate
02	
01	Easy
00	Very Easy

Time

Time simply refers to the period of time (minutes and/or hours) that you perform a cardiovascular exercise activity. The American College of Sports Medicine recommends that you exercise for at least 20 minutes per day, three days per week to achieve any form of cardiovascular system benefit and any metabolism change. If you increase the period of time from 20 minutes to 60 minutes per day, you'll see even greater improvements in caloric expenditure, fat burning, and aerobic capacity.

If you are training for a specific event, you should design a cardiovascular exercise program routine that is specifically tailored to meet the demands of that sport. Refer to the "Personal Fitness Training Program" section on the CD-ROM for more information about cardiovascular training.

Measuring Your Progress

During your fitness program, it is important to measure your progress from time to time. This should help motivate you by showing you just how far you've come, and will also help you determine whether to increase the difficulty level of your fitness program. The best way to measure your progress is to reevaluate your personal fitness assessment test scores (refer to Chapter 3) every three months to update your progress and begin a new personal fitness training program.

Between personal fitness assessment tests, a good way to measure your ongoing progress is to take note of any of the following positive results of your fitness program:

- Your clothes feel looser around your waist line, hips, and thigh areas.

- You have more energy throughout the day.

- You are sleeping better.

- Your resting heart rate measurement has dropped.

- You are breathing easier.

- Your posture has improved.

- You can lift more weight (volume).

Simple improvements like these indicate that your personal fitness training program is improving your overall fitness and health.

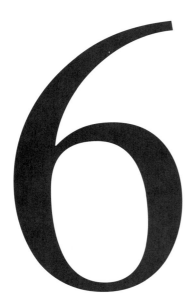

6

General Nutrition

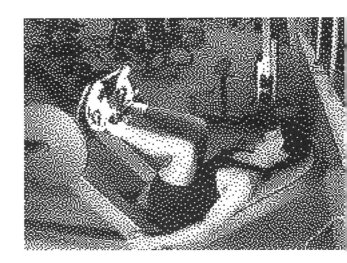

THIS CHAPTER EXPLAINS THE RECOMMENDED DAILY DIETARY HABITS FOR people who are participating in an exercise program. If you want more detailed dietary recommendations—including meals plans and the like—you should get counseling from a registered dietitian for further evaluation and education.

Your nutritional needs will vary depending upon your health and fitness goals. If your aim is to lose body fat, you need to become familiar with the variables that affect weight loss and body fat loss. Above all, you should realize that it's more important to lose body fat than to lose overall body weight. Losing body fat reduces your risk for coronary artery disease, while losing overall body weight doesn't neccessarily reduce this risk. In other words, you shouldn't just cut your calorie intake. Instead you should reduce your intake of fatty foods and increase your physical activity level.

Water

Water is the most essential nutrient your body needs. Forty to sixty percent of your body weight is water. Muscle composition is approximately 70 percent water.

When you exercise, your body loses water through perspiration (dehydration). It is important that you continuously drink water while you are exercising and throughout the day. Eight to ten glasses (8 ounces each) of water are recommended throughout the day for the average person. Your individual level of water intake relates specifically to your body weight, height, and activity levels. Consult a registered dietitian for specific details about your own personal consumption.

Calories

A calorie, or kilocalorie (Kcal), is a measure of heat energy. Food calories supply energy to the body. It is essential that you take in the recommended amount of calories per day. The caloric intake level that's appropriate for you depends on a number of factors, including your height, weight, and gender. If you want to determine a specific figure—that is, approximately how many calories you should consume in a day—again, consult a registered dietitian.

There are three types of calories:

- Carbohydrates

- Fats

- Protein

The American Heart Association recommends a daily total food diet that consists of the following caloric breakdown:

50% carbohydrate

30% fat

20% protein

For individuals who are exercising on a consistent basis, it is recommended that a daily total food diet that consists of the following caloric breakdown:

65% carbohydrate

10% fat

25% protein (2.2 kilograms per pound of body weight)

This caloric breakdown is based upon a higher carbohydrate storage (glycogen storage) that enhances muscular strength, muscular endurance, and athletic performance. The higher level of carbohydrate (65 percent) supplies a greater level of energy to the muscular system. The lower fat level (10 percent) decreases your risk for coronary artery disease. The protein level (25 percent) is increased to offset the body's nitrogen expenditure during intense exercise and to make more amino acids available to the body to help build muscle strength and muscle cell size.

Carbohydrates

Carbohydrate is another term for sugar. Your level of carbohydrate intake will depend upon your desired health and fitness goals.

Carbohydrates come in two forms:

Sucrose (simple sugars)   Simple sugars are used almost immediately during exercise. Examples of simple sugars are processed sugar and fruit sugar.

Glucose (complex sugars)   Complex sugars, also called complex carbohydrates, supply energy to the muscles during exercise. Muscles store large amounts of glucose or glycogen that supply energy to the muscles during prolonged exercise. Complex carbohydrates fuel the body during exercise. Examples of complex sugars are vegetables, bread, pasta, potatoes, and fruit.

Fats

Another term for fat is lipid. High fat intake can lead to obesity, heart disease, heart attacks, and strokes. The lower your level of fat intake, the lower your risk of developing coronary artery disease.

However, fat has positive attributes, too. The body must maintain a certain level of body fat to insulate its inner systems. Like carbohydrates, fat also fuels the body during exercise. Your level of fat intake should depend upon your health and fitness goals.

Examples of foods that are high in fat are cheese, nuts, avocados, cooking oils, and ice cream. It's a good idea to restrict your consumption of these types of foods.

There are three types of fat:

Saturated fat   Saturated fat intake is the most detrimental to the body. Saturated fat has the highest number of fatty acids. It can cause clogged arteries, decreased blood flow transfer, heart attacks, strokes, and other coronary diseases.

Polyunsaturated fat   Polyunsaturated fat has fewer fatty acid molecules than saturated fat, and is therefore better for you than saturated fat. You should have a higher intake of polyunsaturated fat than saturated fat. Polyunsaturated fat is still detrimental to coronary arteries and increases your risk for coronary artery disease.

Monounsaturated fat   Monounsaturated fat has even fewer fatty acid molecules than polyunsaturated fat, and for this reason is the best of all three fats. You should have a higher intake of monounsaturated fat than the other two fats. However, even monounsaturated fat is detrimental to coronary arteries when consumed in excess.

Protein

A protein is composed of amino acids, which help to build muscle mass. The higher your level of muscle mass, the more efficient your basal metabolic rate. An efficient basal metabolic rate, in turn, increases fat and calorie expenditure at a resting state. Your level of protein intake depends upon your desired health and fitness goals; consult with a dietitian to determine your specific protein requirements.

Some foods that are high in protein include egg whites, chicken (white meat), beans, and skim milk.

Vitamins and Minerals

Vitamins and minerals are essential to your daily diet and are found in the natural foods that we consume in our daily diet (fruits, vegetables, meats, and whole grains).

Vitamins are organic compounds (natural and containing carbon) that provide energy to the body, and they are needed in small amounts to assist with chemical reactions within the cells.

Vitamins come in two forms, fat soluble and water soluble. Fat-soluble vitamins (A, D, E, K) are stored in the adipose tissue (fat tissue) and can build up high, and toxic, levels in the body if they are consumed in excess. Water-soluble vitamins (B, C) are not stored in the body, and you should daily consume the vitamins' recommended daily allowances. (Your body excretes unnecessary water-soluble vitamins—but having to continually excrete excessive vitamins can be harmful to your body.)

Minerals are inorganic substances (natural and artificially made) that regulate processes within the body. Minerals are incorporated into different structures within the body to create enzymes, hormones, skeletal bones, skeletal tissues, teeth, and fluids. Calcium and phosphorus are the two most common minerals found in the body. Some of the other prevalent minerals found in the body are iron, zinc, sodium, potassium, magnesium, fluorides, sulfur, copper, and chlorides.

If mineral levels are overabundant in the body, they may cause negative effects. For example, high sodium levels may elevate blood pressure.

Inadequate mineral levels also have negative effects. For example, low iron levels in women can produce anemia. Anemia can restrict oxygen and carbon dioxide removal from the cells. Low calcium levels can facilitate irregular muscle contractions, bone density loss, blood clotting, and improper brain functioning.

For further in-depth information about vitamins and minerals, consult a registered dietitian or your physician.

Recommended Body Fat Levels

Men and women carry fat in different places on their body. Men retain the greatest level of body fat in their abdominal area. Women retain the greatest level of body fat in their hips and thighs. The recommended body fat levels for men and women according to the American College of Sports Medicine are as follows:

	Male	**Female**
Low	6–10% fat	14–18% fat
Optimal	11–17% fat	19–22% fat
Moderate	18–20% fat	23–30% fat
Obesity	Greater than 20% fat	Greater than 30% fat

It's considered unhealthy for men to have a body fat percentage below 3 percent and women to have a body fat percentage below 11 percent. A body fat percentage of over 20 percent for men and over 30 percent for women is also considered unhealthy. Consult Chapter 3 for additional details on having your body fat levels tested.

Body Fat Myths and Misconceptions

There are a number of common myths and misconceptions about body fat. Banish these from your mind if you want to set yourself on a course for greater fitness and health.

Myth number 1 is that fat can be turned into muscle, or vice versa. Muscle is a tissue and fat is a substance. Therefore muscle and fat cannot create one another.

Myth number 2 is that if you weigh more on the scale, you must be overweight. This is untrue. Muscle (lean body mass) weighs approximately 75 percent more than fat. In other words, you can increase your actual body weight without increasing your body fat. You can even increase your body weight and at the same time decrease your percentage of body fat.

Myth number 3 is that weighing yourself on a scale is the best way to determine if you are overweight and have too high a body fat level. In fact, feeling how your clothes fit on your body is a better way to measure body fat loss. You'll also get a better sense of whether you're losing body fat by looking in the mirror with no clothes on.

Physical Activity Levels for Body Fat and Weight Loss

The amount of physical exercise you get has a profound effect upon your level of body fat. If you increase your physical activity level, you will expend greater amounts of calories and fat, depending upon how long and at what level of intensity you exercise (expending 3,500 calories burns up one pound of fat). Here are some general guidelines:

- Consistent aerobic/cardiovascular exercise (20 minutes, three times per week) will improve your cardiovascular system, increase your metabolism, and burn body fat and calories. For additional details on cardiovascular training routines that will suit your needs, refer to the "Personal Fitness Training Program" section on the CD-ROM.

- Consistent weight/strength training (20 minutes, three times per week) will increase your muscular strength, enhance your muscular endurance, result in a leaner body mass, and favorable affect your bone density. For in-depth cover of strength training routines, refer to the "Personal Fitness Training Program" section on the CD-ROM

■ Stretching before and after exercise will increase the range of motion of your joints and muscles. Increasing your flexibility also decreases your risk of injury while exercising. For descriptions of various stretching exercises, refer to the "Personal Fitness Training Program" section on the CD-ROM.

The following list points out the levels of risk for gaining body fat and overall body weight due to insufficient caloric expenditure. (This list includes the number of calories you expend as part of your basal metabolic rate with activity.)

Optimal	5,000 Kcals per week
Moderate	500-5,000 Kcals per week
Obesity	Fewer than 500 Kcals per week

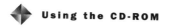
Using the CD-ROM

This CD-ROM will work with both Macintosh and PC computers running Windows. To launch *Your Personal Fitness Trainer* on a Macintosh,

1. If you do not have QuickTime installed, drag and drop it into your system folder, then restart your machine.

2. Double-click on the Trainer icon in the PFT™ window.

To lauch *Your Personal Fitness Trainer* on a PC,

1. If you currently have a version of QuickTime installed, please remove it using the Drivers control panel in Windows.

2. Double-click on the TRAINER.EXE icon in the File Manager.

For best results, one of the video and sound cards listed below should be installed in your computer. The following table lists cards that have been tested and that offer optimum viewing of the CD-ROM.

VIDEO CARDS		DRIVER	
	Bus	**Date**	**Rev**
Actix ProStar VL	VLB	8/18/93	1.42
ATI Graphics Ultra	ISA	3/19/93	2.3
ATI Graphis Ultra Plus	ISA	4/25/94	2.3
ATI Graphics Ultra Pro	VLB	4/25/94	2.3
ATI Graphics Ultra Pro	ISA	4/25/94	2.3
Blackship Color Designer	VLB	7/8/93	1.32
Diamond Speed Star Pro	ISA	2/17/94	1.08
Diamond Speed Star VGA	ISA	4/14/92	
Diamond Stealth 24	VLB	6/3/94	3.0
Diamond Stealth Pro	VLB	10/6/93	
ELSA Winner2000 Pro	PCI	6/23/94	1.22
Hercules Dynamite Pro	ISA	12/1/93	2.10
Hercules Dynamite Pro	VLB	12/1/93	3.0
Hercules Graphite Power	ISA	4/6/94	2.10
IBM XGA Display	MCA	11/12/93	2.11
Matrox MGA Power Graphics	PCI	3/28/93	1.42
Media Vision ProGraphics 1280	VLB	9/15/93	1.01
Media Vision ProGraphics1024	VLB	4/15/94	1.5

VIDEO CARDS		DRIVER	
	Bus	Date	Rev
Mitac MVA-CL5428-1MB	VLB	3/15/94	1.43
Number Nine 9GXe Level 10	ISA	2/9/94	3.11
Number Nine 9GXe Level 11	VLB	2/9/94	3.10
Number Nine 9GXe Level 14	VLB	4/7/94	3.15
Number Nine 9GXE64	VLB	6/22/94	1.19.04
Orchid Celsius	VLB	10/1/93	1.32
Orchid Fahrenheit 1280 Plus	VLB	3/1/94	7
Orchid Fahrenheit VA	VLB	4/29/93	5.01
Orchid Kelvin 64	PCI	3/14/94	1.1
Orchid Kelvin 64	VLB	2/23/94	1.21
Orchid ProDesigner IIS	ISA	3/1/92	2.0
Paradise WD90c33	VLB	6/28/93	1.2
Standard 1Mb-24X	ISA	3/19/93	1.30
STB Horizon VL Pro	VLB	6/29/93	1.3
STB Lightspeed	PCI	12/1/93	1.1
STB Pegasus	VLB	11/29/93	1.3
TrueVision Bravado 9	ISA	1/15/92	

SOUND CARDS

Sound Card

Compaq Business Audio

Creative Labs SoundBlaster

Creative Labs SoundBlaster Pro

Creative Labs SoundBlaster 16

Creative Labs SoundBlaster AWE32

Gateway 2000

IBM M-Audio

MediaVision ProAudio Spectrum

MediaVision ProAudio Spectrum 16

MediaVision ProAudio Spectrum 16 Pro

MicroSoft SoundSystem Version 1

MicroSoft SoundSystem Version 2

Orchid SoundWave 32

Reveal Forte 16

Roland Rap-10